Multiple Sclerosis:
A Neuropsychiatric
Disorder

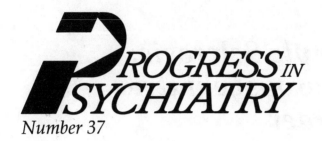

Number 37

David Spiegel, M.D.
Series Editor

Multiple Sclerosis: A Neuropsychiatric Disorder

Edited by
Uriel Halbreich, M.D.

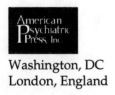
American
Psychiatric
Press, Inc

Washington, DC
London, England

Note: The authors have worked to ensure that all information in this book concerning drug dosages, schedules, and routes of administration is accurate as of the time of publication and consistent with standards set by the U.S. Food and Drug Administration and the general medical community. As medical research and practice advance, however, therapeutic standards may change. For this reason and because human and mechanical errors sometimes occur, we recommend that readers follow the advice of a physician who is directly involved in their care or the care of a member of their family.

Books published by the American Psychiatric Press, Inc., represent the views and opinions of the individual authors and do not necessarily represent the policies and opinions of the Press or the American Psychiatric Association.

Copyright © 1993 American Psychiatric Press, Inc.
ALL RIGHTS RESERVED
Manufactured in the United States of America on acid-free paper
First Edition   96 95 94 93   4 3 2 1

American Psychiatric Press, Inc.
1400 K Street, N.W., Washington, DC   20005

Library of Congress Cataloging-in-Publication Data

Multiple sclerosis : a neuropsychiatric disorder / edited by Uriel
   Halbreich. — 1st ed.
      p. cm. — (Progress in psychiatry series ; no. 37)
   Includes bibliographical references and index.
   ISBN 0-88048-463-2 (alk. paper)
      1. Multiple sclerosis—Psychological aspects. 2. Neuropsychiatry.
I. Halbreich, Uriel, 1943–   . II. Series: Progress in psychiatry
series ; #37.
      [DNLM: 1. Affective Disorders—etiology. 2. Multiple Sclerosis.
3. Neuropsychology.   WL 360 M95634]
RC377.M8433 1993
616.8'34—dc20
DNLM/DLC
for Library of Congress   92-22041
                                                                      CIP

British Library Cataloguing in Publication Data
A CIP record is available from the British Library.

Contents

Contributors

Carol M. Brownscheidle, Ph.D.
Clinical Assistant Professor, Department of Rehabilitation Medicine, School of Medicine and Biomedical Sciences, State University of New York at Buffalo, Buffalo, New York

Carl V. Granger, M.D.
Professor of Rehabilitation Medicine; Director, Center for Functional Assessment Research, Department of Rehabilitation Medicine; Co-Director, University at Buffalo Multiple Sclerosis System, School of Medicine and Biomedical Sciences, State University of New York at Buffalo, Buffalo, New York

Igor Grant, M.D., F.R.C.P.C.
Professor and Vice Chairman, Department of Psychiatry, University of California, San Diego, San Diego, California

Uriel Halbreich, M.D.
Professor of Psychiatry, Research Professor of Obstetrics and Gynecology, Director of Biobehavioral Research, School of Medicine and Biomedical Sciences, State University of New York at Buffalo, Buffalo, New York

Margaret M. Hens, M.S., R.N.
Director of Patient Care, Bernard B. Hoffman Multiple Sclerosis Center, University at Buffalo Multiple Sclerosis System, School of Medicine and Biomedical Sciences, State University of New York at Buffalo, Buffalo, New York

Lawrence Jacobs, M.D.
Professor of Neurology, School of Medicine and Biomedical Sciences, State University of New York at Buffalo; Head, Department of Neurology, Buffalo General Hospital; Chief, The Baird Multiple Sclerosis Center, Millard Fillmore Hospital, Buffalo, New York

Roland Martin, M.D.
Visiting Fellow, Neuroimmunology Branch, National
Institute of Neurological Disorders and Stroke, Bethesda,
Maryland

Henry F. McFarland, M.D.
Deputy Chief, Neuroimmunology Branch, National
Institute of Neurological Disorders and Stroke, Bethesda,
Maryland

Sarah L. Minden, M.D.
Instructor in Psychiatry, Harvard Medical School; Division
of Psychiatry, Brigham and Women's Hospital, Boston,
Massachusetts

Frederick E. Munschauer, M.D.
Assistant Professor of Neurology, State University of New
York at Buffalo; Attending Neurologist, Department of
Neurology, Buffalo General Hospital and The Baird
Multiple Sclerosis Center, Millard Fillmore Hospital,
Buffalo, New York

Patrick Pullicino, M.D.
Assistant Professor of Neurology, State University of New
York at Buffalo; Attending Neurologist, Buffalo General
Hospital and The Baird Multiple Sclerosis Center, Millard
Fillmore Hospital, Buffalo, New York

Stephen M. Rao, Ph.D.
Professor of Neurology, Section of Neuropsychology,
Medical College of Wisconsin, Milwaukee, Wisconsin

Stephen C. Reingold, Ph.D.
Vice President, Research and Medical Programs, The
National Multiple Sclerosis Society, New York, New York

Lawrence M. Samkoff, M.D.
Assistant Professor of Neurology, Medical Rehabilitation
Research and Training Center for Multiple Sclerosis, Albert
Einstein College of Medicine, Bronx, New York

Labe C. Scheinberg, M.D.
Professor of Neurology, Psychiatry and Rehabilitation
Department of Neurology, Albert Einstein College of
Medicine, Bronx, New York

Randolph B. Schiffer, M.D.
Associate Professor of Neurology and Psychiatry,
University of Rochester, School of Medicine and Dentistry;
Associated Chairman for Clinical Affairs, Departments of
Neurology and Psychiatry, Strong Memorial Hospital,
Rochester, New York

Charles R. Smith, M.D.
Assistant Professor of Neurology, Medical Rehabilitation
Research and Training Center for Multiple Sclerosis, Albert
Einstein College of Medicine, Bronx, New York

Introduction to the Progress in Psychiatry Series

The Progress in Psychiatry Series is designed to capture in print the excitement that comes from assembling a diverse group of experts from various locations to examine in detail the newest information about a developing aspect of psychiatry. This series emerged as a collaboration between the American Psychiatric Association's (APA) Scientific Program Committee and the American Psychiatric Press, Inc. Great interest is generated by a number of the symposia presented each year at the APA annual meeting, and we realized that much of the information presented there, carefully assembled by people who are deeply immersed in a given area, would unfortunately not appear together in print. The symposia sessions at the annual meetings provide an unusual opportunity for experts who otherwise might not meet on the same platform to share their diverse viewpoints for a period of 3 hours. Some new themes are repeatedly reinforced and gain credence, while in other instances disagreements emerge, enabling the audience and now the reader to reach informed decisions about new directions in the field. The Progress in Psychiatry Series allows us to publish and capture some of the best of the symposia and thus provide an in-depth treatment of specific areas that might not otherwise be presented in broader review formats.

Psychiatry is by nature an interface discipline, combining the study of mind and brain, of individual and social environments, of the humane and the scientific. Therefore, progress in the field is rarely linear—it often comes from unexpected sources. Further, new developments emerge from an array of viewpoints that do not necessarily provide immediate agreement but rather expert examination of the issues. We intend to present innovative ideas and data that will enable you, the reader, to participate in this process.

We believe the Progress in Psychiatry Series will provide you with an opportunity to review timely new information in specific fields of interest as they are developing. We hope you find that the excitement of the presentations is captured in the written word and that this book proves to be informative and enjoyable reading.

David Spiegel, M.D.
Series Editor
Progress in Psychiatry Series

Progress in Psychiatry Series Titles

The Borderline: Current Empirical Research (#1)
Edited by Thomas H. McGlashan, M.D.

Premenstrual Syndrome: Current Findings and Future Directions (#2)
Edited by Howard J. Osofsky, M.D., Ph.D.,
and Susan J. Blumenthal, M.D.

Treatment of Affective Disorders in the Elderly (#3)
Edited by Charles A. Shamoian, M.D.

Post-Traumatic Stress Disorder in Children (#4)
Edited by Spencer Eth, M.D., and Robert S. Pynoos, M.D., M.P.H.

The Psychiatric Implications of Menstruation (#5)
Edited by Judith H. Gold, M.D., F.R.C.P.C.

Can Schizophrenia Be Localized in the Brain? (#6)
Edited by Nancy C. Andreasen, M.D., Ph.D.

Medical Mimics of Psychiatric Disorders (#7)
Edited by Irl Extein, M.D., and Mark S. Gold, M.D.

Biopsychosocial Aspects of Bereavement (#8)
Edited by Sidney Zisook, M.D.

Psychiatric Pharmacosciences of Children and Adolescents (#9)
Edited by Charles Popper, M.D.

Psychobiology of Bulimia (#10)
Edited by James I. Hudson, M.D., and Harrison G. Pope, Jr., M.D.

Cerebral Hemisphere Function in Depression (#11)
Edited by Marcel Kinsbourne, M.D.

Eating Behavior in Eating Disorders (#12)
Edited by B. Timothy Walsh, M.D.

Tardive Dyskinesia: Biological Mechanisms and Clinical Aspects (#13)
Edited by Marion E. Wolf, M.D., and Aron D. Mosnaim, Ph.D.

Current Approaches to the Prediction of Violence (#14)
Edited by David A. Brizer, M.D., and Martha L. Crowner, M.D.

Treatment of Tricyclic-Resistant Depression (#15)
Edited by Irl L. Extein, M.D.

Depressive Disorders and Immunity (#16)
Edited by Andrew H. Miller, M.D.

Depression and Families: Impact and Treatment (#17)
Edited by Gabor I. Keitner, M.D.

Depression in Schizophrenia (#18)
Edited by Lynn E. DeLisi, M.D.

Biological Assessment and Treatment of Posttraumatic Stress Disorder (#19)
Edited by Earl L. Giller, Jr., M.D., Ph.D.

Personality Disorders: New Perspectives on Diagnostic Validity (#20)
Edited by John M. Oldham, M.D.

Serotonin in Major Psychiatric Disorders (#21)
Edited by Emil F. Coccaro, M.D., and Dennis L. Murphy, M.D.

Amino Acids in Psychiatric Disease (#22)
Edited by Mary Ann Richardson, Ph.D.

Family Environment and Borderline Personality Disorder (#23)
Edited by Paul Skevington Links, M.D.

Biological Rhythms, Mood Disorders, Light Therapy, and the Pineal Gland (#24)
Edited by Mohammad Shafii, M.D.,
and Sharon Lee Shafii, R.N., B.S.N.

Treatment Strategies for Refractory Depression (#25)
Edited by Steven P. Roose, M.D.,
and Alexander H. Glassman, M.D.

Combination Pharmacotherapy and Psychotherapy for Depression (#26)
Edited by Donna Manning, M.D., and Allen J. Frances, M.D.

The Neuroleptic Nonresponsive Patient: Characterization and Treatment (#27)
Edited by Burt Angrist, M.D., and S. Charles Schulz, M.D.

Negative Schizophrenic Symptoms: Pathophysiology and Clinical Implications (#28)
Edited by John F. Greden, M.D., and Rajiv Tandon, M.D.

Neuropeptides and Psychiatric Disorders (#29)
Edited by Charles B. Nemeroff, M.D., Ph.D.

Central Nervous System Peptide Mechanisms in Stress and Depression (#30)
Edited by S. Craig Risch, M.D.

Current Concepts of Somatization: Research and Clinical Perspectives (#31)
Edited by Laurence J. Kirmayer, M.D., F.R.C.P.C., and James M. Robbins, Ph.D.

Mental Retardation: Developing Pharmacotherapies (#32)
Edited by John J. Ratey, M.D.

Positron-Emission Tomography in Schizophrenia Research (#33)
Edited by Nora D. Volkow, M.D., and Alfred P. Wolf, Ph.D.

Brain Imaging in Affective Disorders (#34)
Edited by Peter Hauser, M.D.

Psychoimmunology Update (#35)
Edited by Jack M. Gorman, M.D., and Robert M. Kertzner, M.D.

Biology of Anxiety Disorders (#36)
Edited by Rudolf Hoehn-Saric, M.D., and Daniel R. McLeod, Ph.D.

Multiple Sclerosis: A Neuropsychiatric Disorder (#37)
Edited by Uriel Halbreich, M.D.

Introduction

Multiple sclerosis (MS) is quite a prevalent disease that causes disability and agony. Close examination shows that substantial progress has been achieved in our knowledge of MS in the last 10 years. It also clearly demonstrates the realistic hope for further achievements in our understanding of the genetics and pathophysiology of MS as well as in the diagnosis, treatment, and rehabilitation of patients with this disease.

This book was written by an interdisciplinary group. We hope that together we provide an updated picture of the state of the art in research, as well as solid clinical information. This book focuses on a disease, but this disease seriously affects individual patients and their families. Therefore, this book is designed so that much of the scientifically accurate information will be of interest and help to people at different levels, including scientists and clinician-specialists, primary care physicians who first encounter the patient and have to determine the different diagnosis, and last, but not least, the patients and their families who are anxious to know "what's going on."

The message that we hope to convey in this book is that MS is a neurostructural neuropsychiatric disorder with diversified clinical features that should be differentiated from other disseminated neurostructural disorders. Depression and other mood and behavioral changes are quite prevalent in patients with MS, as is cognitive impairment. The specific symptoms of MS are probably associated with the location and overall magnitude of the lesions. Genetic and family components probably play a role in the vulnerability to develop the autoimmune pathogenesis of MS, but specific episodes might be precipitated or exacerbated by stressful life events.

Because MS affects patients and their families and causes a disability, rehabilitation plays a significant role in each patient's life. Although various effective treatment modalities are currently applied, it seems that attempts at tackling the autoimmune pathological processes are increasingly taking a central stage in this arena. In the background, the National Association of Multiple Sclerosis is an example par excellence of the constructive and stimulating role that patients' advocacy groups can play in the advancement of knowledge and management of such a prevalent disorder.

In this volume, the clinical features of MS are described in Chapter 1 by Smith, Samkoff, and Scheinberg from the Albert Einstein College of Medicine. They emphasize the diagnostic process of the disorder and assess the value of diagnostic tests that might add to the establishment of diagnosis. MS should be distinguished from other neurostructural disorders, therefore the differential diagnosis of MS is of utmost importance, especially because of the varied and diversified clinical manifestations. As the authors put it, "There still remains no substitute for a careful history, thorough examination, and sound clinical judgment."

In Chapter 2, Minden, of Harvard Medical School, and Schiffer, of the University of Rochester, New York, focus on depression and other affective disorders in MS. Depression, euphoria, indifference, and other mood and cognitive disorders are among the most noticeable characteristics of MS. They are heuristically intriguing because they might provide some insight into the association between specific mental symptoms and specific localized pathological processes in the brain. Clinically they are challenging because not all depressed MS patients receive adequate psychiatric treatment. Furthermore, some symptoms (e.g., indifference and euphoria) raise ethical issues, such as whether they should be treated at all because such symptoms might actually play a positive role in patients' interaction with their environment.

Rao, from the Medical College of Wisconsin, has been investigating the possible association between location of MS plaques and cognitive impairment. In Chapter 3, he discusses how even though cognitive dysfunctions can have a significant impact on patients' quality of life, unfortunately very little attention has been devoted to the treatment of these disorders. A first step in that direction is further elucidation of the pathophysiology of their symptoms. With the available imaging techniques, we may already have tools for such studies. Substantial progress in the understanding and eventual treatment of cognitive dysfunctions in patients with MS and other related disorders can be reasonably anticipated.

A real breakthrough in the understanding of MS will hopefully be provided by the efforts in molecular biology and immunology. In Chapter 4, Martin and McFarland, of the Neuroimmunology Branch of the National Institute of Neurological Disorders and Stroke, present the case for genetic transmittal of MS, which might be different within and across patients, especially for different ethnic groups. The putative genes for MS probably play a role in the autoimmune pathogenesis of the disorder. Martin and McFarland present a compelling argument that the recent astounding progress in the development of genetic probes and mapping techniques, in combination with the advances in clinical diagnosis, will lead to the determination of the genetic links of MS that will give the needed clue to its causes.

As is the case with any disorder, the most important *practical* questions about MS are "What is the treatment?" and "How effective is it?" In Chapter 5, Jacobs, Munschauer, and Pullicino, of the State University of New York at Buffalo, argue that the most effective and promising modes of treatment of MS are those that interfere with abnormalities of the immune system. The response to treatment trials supports the assertion that autoimmune abnormalities are a pivotal process in the pathogenesis of MS. Immunosuppression by adrenocoritcotropic hormone (ACTH), steroids, cyclophosphamide, azathioprine, and other agents has been shown to be quite effective, especially for chronic progressive MS. Recently, interferon-β has been introduced on an experimental basis and is quite a promising treatment modality. These developments might be an indication that we are moving toward more specific interventions as treatment for specific immune defects in MS.

The genetic and immune aspects of MS provide only a partial view of the MS story. In Chapter 6, Grant, of the University of California, San Diego, underscores the importance of the environment, stress, and other psychosocial factors in the onset, development, exacerbations, course, and phenomenology of MS. The psychosocial aspects of MS also influence treatment responses. It has been demonstrated that adaptational and coping styles influence the quality of life and well-being of patients.

Furthermore, MS patients with a solid social support network are clinically better than those who receive the same pharmacological treatment but do not enjoy the same reliable and warm support.

This issue is very important in a disease that causes such a significant chronic disability. In Chapter 7, Granger, Hens, and Brownscheidle, of the Department of Rehabilitation Medicine of the State University of New York at Buffalo, review the disability aspects of MS and the ways to assess their nature and their severity. Based on their experience at Buffalo, the authors discuss the detailed procedures needed. Each individual patient needs a detailed functional assessment, and treatment strategy should be developed and tailored to measure according to actual functions impaired. The authors also provide recommendations for rehabilitation treatment for MS.

A crucial role in the progress toward better understanding, treatment, and rehabilitation of patients with MS is played by the patients themselves, as well as their advocacy groups and support associations. Reingold, the author of Chapter 8, is the Vice President for Research and Medical Programs of the National Multiple Sclerosis Society, which represents over 170,000 individuals with MS and exercises significant influence on research and public policy related to MS and other chronic disabilities. The Society is an exemplary bridge between people with MS, the scientific and clinical communities, and the political and financial systems. Its fund-raising, research support, and educational activities and services emphasize the commitment of all people and disciplines involved.

The interdisciplinary effort and the alliance between scientists, clinicians, and patients represented in this book will hopefully lead to further heuristic scientific advances and better well-being of patients. Many of the concepts presented here can be generalized and/or adapted to other neurostructural disorders. Hopefully they will.

Uriel Halbreich, M.D.

Chapter 1

Clinical Features, Assessment, and Differential Diagnosis of Multiple Sclerosis

Charles R. Smith, M.D., Lawrence M. Samkoff, M.D., and Labe C. Scheinberg, M.D.

Multiple sclerosis (MS) is the most common of the neurological diseases characterized pathologically by central nervous system (CNS) demyelination. Despite decades of intensive scientific study, neither the cause nor the pathogenesis of MS is known, and the disease remains very much a mystery. However, its impact is obvious and can hardly be overstated. In the United States, MS is a major cause of severe disability in the young adult population. Consequently, the burden on society in terms of both human suffering and economic losses is enormous. For example, it has been estimated that the total economic burden of MS in the United States may amount to as much as $15,000 per year for each family. Total current and future lifetime costs to society may approach $29 billion (Inman 1984). The physical and psychological effects of an unpredictable disease with a wide range of clinical expression strain relationships both at home and the workplace and test the ability of even the most dedicated health care provider to deal with its widespread ramifications. In this chapter, we review the salient clinical features of MS, including the epidemiology, pathogenesis, symptoms, prognosis, diagnosis, and differential diagnosis of MS. In the discussion of symptoms, we focus not only on the important neurological complaints, but also include a review of the important medical and psychosocial complications.

This work was supported in part by The National Institute on Disability and Rehabilitation Research Grant #133B80018.

EPIDEMIOLOGY

The most recent epidemiological studies for MS in the United States suggest an incidence rate as high as 6.3 per 100,000 and a prevalence rate as high as 177 per 100,000 (see Wynn et al. 1990). These figures represent a substantial increase in the numbers of cases over those reported only a few years ago. Based on a total population of 250 million, they suggest an estimated MS population of about 240,000 people in the United States. Even these figures likely represent a substantial underestimate of the true incidence and prevalence of MS, for several reasons. First, patients with minor neurological symptoms may never seek neurological attention, and many physicians are unwilling to consider the diagnosis in patients with minimal findings. There are also many reports of MS as an incidental finding at autopsy when review of the clinical records indicates no suggestion of disease expression during life (Gilbert and Sadler 1983; Phadke and Best 1983). Finally, even the most recent studies are based on data collected before the extensive use of newer, more sensitive diagnostic tests such as magnetic resonance imaging (MRI). Consequently, some suspect that the true prevalence of MS may be much greater than that now reported (D. W. Anderson et al. 1992).

PATHOGENESIS

MS is primarily a disease of white females: the female to male ratio and the white to black ratio are both nearly 2:1 (Kurtzke et al. 1979). Although more than 90% of patients initially present between the ages of 10 and 60 years, the peak age at onset is in the fourth decade. Occurrence before age 10 is very rare, but as many as 7% of cases present with their first symptoms after age 60 (Baum and Rothschild 1981).

Although the cause is unknown, current evidence suggests that MS is an autoimmune disease precipitated by an environmental agent in a genetically predisposed individual. The autoimmune contention is based on several lines of evidence including the presence of immune cells at the sites of active demyelination (Traugott et al. 1983), a variety of peripheral blood

immune abnormalities (Hafler and Weiner 1989), and close similarities of MS to the experimental autoimmune animal disease,
experimental allergic encephalomyelitis (Lassmann 1983). That
MS is probably precipitated by an environmental agent is suggested by epidemiological studies that indicate a substantially
higher prevalence of the disease in the temperate and colder
regions of the world (Kurtzke 1983a). Studies of migrating humans have also shown that the chance of getting MS is determined by geographic residence before middle adolescence (Elian
and Dean 1987; Visscher et al. 1977). Finally, there have been
several well-studied "epidemics" of MS such as the one that
occurred on the Faeroe Islands (Kurtzke 1977). The evidence
supports the concept of an age-specific vulnerability to an un-
identified environmental agent. Although a virus or perhaps a
combination of viruses has long been considered the most likely
precipitant of MS, no direct evidence for a viral cause has ever
been substantiated.

Although the disease is not inherited, there appears to be a
genetic predisposition to MS. As many as 15% of MS patients
have a first-degree relative also carrying the diagnosis (Sadovnick and Baird 1988). Twin studies have demonstrated that
monozygotic twins have a concordance rate of 26%, whereas
fraternal twins have a concordance rate of about 2%, which is not
significantly different from the concordance in nontwin siblings
(Ebers et al. 1986). Certain human leukocyte antigens (HLAs) are
known to be more highly represented in populations of MS patients, depending on ethnicity. For patients of Northern European and North American heritage, they include HLA-A3, -B7,
-Dw2, and -DR2. More recent findings linking certain histocompatibility factors and T-cell receptor genes have provided new
insights that may relate to disease susceptibility (Beall et al. 1989).

SYMPTOMS

The symptoms of MS can be conveniently categorized as primary, secondary, or tertiary. The primary symptoms reflect the
strategic effects of a discrete plaque of demyelination on neurological function. Examples include monocular visual loss from
optic neuritis, incontinence of urine from myelopathy, and inten-

tion tremor from demyelination of the cerebellar outflow tracts. The secondary symptoms are the nonneurological complications that ensue directly as a consequence of the primary ones and include urinary tract infection because of urinary retention, pressure sores because of immobility, and aspiration pneumonia because of dysphagia. Finally, the tertiary symptoms are the psychological, social, and vocational ramifications of the disease on the patient, family, and community.

For many patients, attention to all three categories of symptoms is necessary to provide optimal rehabilitation and to prevent complications. Consequently, the needs of patients, especially for those most severely affected, are best served in a comprehensive care setting in which a team approach can be coordinated. Team members include neurologists, specialized nurses, occupational and physical therapists, social workers, and psychologists. There must be an established working relationship with other medical practitioners such as internists, physiatrists, urologists, orthopedists, and psychiatrists to assist when special needs arise. The center must coordinate care so that the patients' needs are satisfied by those most familiar with the ramifications of the disease. Otherwise, care becomes fractionated, and unnecessary complications ensue.

Primary Symptoms

When asked to list their primary complaints, patients will frequently cite gait difficulties and impaired bladder control. This should not be surprising because the lesions of MS are scattered in the white matter of the CNS and those neurological functions served by the longest pathways are most likely to be involved. The other most frequently cited symptoms are constipation, sexual dysfunction, visual impairment, and fatigue.

Gait. Symptoms resulting in altered gait include weakness, stiffness, heaviness, imbalance, and numbness or, as is most often the case, a combination of these. Neurological examination discloses paralysis, spasticity, cerebellar ataxia, or sensory loss, any or all of which in combination may be responsible for the symptoms. Not infrequently, complaints are referable to only one lower limb, but bilateral findings on examination are the rule.

In the earliest phases of gait impairment, patients may complain of easy fatigability or difficulty with running. If the symptoms progress, they may note dragging of one or both lower limbs, frequently precipitated by prolonged exercise. Symptoms may fluctuate throughout the day and may worsen under conditions of high ambient temperature. Equilibrium may be defective, and falling is frequent. Patients become more dependent on the handrails of staircases and must frequently stop and rest when walking any distance. If the disease is progressive, independent gait may become hazardous, and gait aids become necessary. Unfortunately for some, gait becomes impossible, even with aids, and the use of a wheelchair becomes inevitable.

Careful evaluation of the history and physical examination is necessary to correctly identify the precise mechanism of abnormal gait. For example, patients with symptomatic spasticity may also report spasms of the lower limbs, which may be painful and may occur at night, interfering with sleep. Both weakness and spasticity can produce complaints of "heaviness" or "dragging," but spastic patients may additionally describe their lower limbs as being "stiff." Physical examination discloses which of these are present and gives an estimate of the relative contribution of each to the complaint.

Cerebellar disturbances are among the most common symptoms of MS, and cerebellar ataxia is probably the most frequent finding responsible for gait complaints. Patients describe losing their balance, especially on turning. On examination, most patients will have at least some difficulty with tandem gait. Although patients frequently have findings suggesting abnormal dorsal column function in the lower limbs, such as impaired vibratory or position sense, sensory ataxia seems only infrequently to be a primary cause of imbalance or gait impairment.

Bladder, bowel, and sexual dysfunction. Urinary symptoms occur in the majority of MS patients and are typically conjoined with bowel and sexual complaints. "Irritative" urinary symptoms indicating uninhibited detrusor contractions include urgency, frequency, nocturia, and urgency incontinence; complaints suggestive of urinary retention include weak urinary stream, incomplete emptying with "double voiding," and spontaneous interruptions of the urinary stream. Any of these symptoms may occur in combination. Consequently, attempting to deduce the nature of the disturbance based on history alone frequently yields inaccurate conclusions and, thus, errors in treatment (Blaivas et al. 1984).

Quite simply, urinary symptoms directly resulting from the neurological lesions of MS can be categorized as failure to store urine or failure to empty the bladder and may occur in combination (Blaivas 1979). Patients with failure to store have a small-capacity bladder with involuntary detrusor contractions. Patients with failure to empty may have either detrusor paralysis, which is uncommon in MS, or outlet obstruction because of detrusor-external sphincter dyssynergia (DESD) (Blaivas et al. 1981a). DESD results from the failure to coordinate detrusor contraction with external urinary sphincter relaxation and always signifies a lesion above the sacral segments of the spinal cord but below the pontine reticular formation, the site of an important facilitatory center for bladder reflexes (Blaivas et al. 1981b). The result is obstruction of urinary flow and an elevated residual urine, predisposing to urinary tract infection. Therefore, when there are urinary complaints, the goals of intervention are threefold: 1) to identify complicating urinary tract infection, 2) to prevent further complications, and 3) to control symptoms. Consequently, a microscopic urinalysis and culture of urine should be obtained on the first evaluation or if there is any subsequent change in symptoms. A postvoiding residual urine should be determined on all patients with urinary symptoms before initiating treatment so that correct therapy may be given.

Bowel complaints are at least as common as urinary symptoms, the most frequent complaint being constipation (Glick et al. 1982). Although constipation may be attributed directly to the effects of the neurological lesions on bowel motility, other factors such as diet, fluid intake, and medications may be important contributing factors. It should be remembered that many patients control irritative urinary symptoms by reducing fluid intake. Less frequently, stool incontinence may occur. Diarrhea is not a symptom of MS and should suggest another problem, such as spurious diarrhea because of fecal impaction (Levine 1985).

Sexual complaints are probably as frequent as bladder and bowel symptoms. This should not be surprising as all three functions are likely subserved by similar spinal pathways. The most frequent complaint of males is impotence; for women it is decreased libido (Barrett 1977). Sexual problems may relate to the psychological ramifications of the disease, as well as to the effects of the neurological lesions (Kalb et al. 1987). For many, both factors contribute, an important fact when considering treatment. Furthermore, many medications can interfere with sexual responses and may contribute to the problem.

Sensory problems. Sensory symptoms are nearly universal in MS, but because confirmatory findings are not always present such complaints are often ignored by physicians. This may be particularly problematic for patients in the early stages of their disease, when there are no other symptoms or definite objective findings on physical examination. Not uncommonly, patients are given psychiatric diagnoses when no physical cause can be found for their complaints. Compounding the problem, sensory complaints are often complicated and inexactly described. When the dorsal columns are involved, sensations may be variously described as "vibration," "bands," "tingling," or "pins and needles." Such sensations can affect an entire limb or several limbs or may encircle specific areas of a limb or the trunk. Symptoms referable to the spinothalamic pathways are typically uncomfortable and frequently painful. Although a popular misconception, pain is not rare in MS (Clifford and Trotter 1984). Occasionally, abnormal sensations may adopt a clearly dermatomal distribution suggesting demyelination at the dorsal root entry zone at the corresponding level of the spinal cord. Consequently, it may be difficult to determine through history and physical examination whether radicular pain is caused by MS or another unrelated condition such as a herniated intervertebral disk.

Probably, the most common sensory finding in MS is impaired vibratory sense of the distal lower limbs. Although uncommon, a rather characteristic sensory syndrome is the sensory useless hand, which may be bilateral. Patients have severe sensory impairment, and the abnormalities on physical examination suggest primarily dorsal column involvement. Fortunately, most patients recover completely from this otherwise very disabling but typically short-lived phenomenon. Another characteristic sign of dorsal column involvement in MS is Lhermitte's sign, in which the patient experiences a sensation of tingling down the back and possibly the extremities when the head is flexed forward.

Upper-extremities problems.   Many patients have symptoms referable to the upper limbs. Upper-limb problems include weakness, clumsiness, tremor, and numbness. Initially, difficulty with tasks requiring fine motor control, such as doing up buttons or writing, are described. Corticospinal, dorsal column, or cerebellar involvement may be responsible for impaired digital dexterity as can be observed when patients are asked to execute these movements. When severe, involvement of the upper limbs can have a devastating impact because patients may become totally dependent on others for all activities of daily living.

Vision.   Visual complaints are very characteristic and result either from lesions of the optic nerves or from the pathways subserving extraocular muscle movements. Although visual acuity—as measured by standard instruments, such as the Snellen chart—may seem quite normal, complaints may reflect defective contrast sensitivity or color perception, which are not always evaluated. Ocular motility problems may produce a variety of complaints including oscillopsia (especially when there is primary position oscillatory nystagmus) and blurred vision without diplopia (e.g., from internuclear ophthalmoplegia). Frank diplopia may occur but tends to be transient. The most frequent cause of frank diplopia is involvement of the sixth cranial nerve fibers as they course through the brain stem.

Brain stem dysfunction.   Other complaints that can be frequently ascribed to brain stem dysfunction include dysarthria and dysphagia. Many patients with dysarthria have cerebellar causes for speech impairment, although pseudobulbar palsy from bilateral corticobulbar involvement also occurs. Patients with cerebellar speech disturbances may have nystagmus and intention tremor of the limbs (Charcot's triad). Dysphagia is a potentially serious complication of MS because it can lead to aspiration. In fact, aspiration pneumonia is one of the most common causes of death among MS patients, when the cause of death can be directly attributed to the disease. Trigeminal neuralgia is another manifestation of brain stem involvement; when it occurs in a young person, it is nearly diagnostic of MS. Otherwise, typical Bell's palsy is said to occur in about 5% of cases and is thought to be caused by demyelination at the root exit zone of the facial nerve if not conjoined with lateral rectus palsy. Symptomatic hearing loss is distinctly rare, although audiometry frequently discloses subtle asymptomatic abnormalities (Daugherty et al. 1983). Finally, facial myokymia—an involuntary, rapid-flickering movement of the facial muscles without weakness—is a frequent finding but is often unnoticed by patients.

Dementia. Dementia is not as rare in MS as was previously believed. Studies (Peyser et al. 1980; Rao et al. 1984) have shown that about 50% of MS patients have intellectual impairment, as measured by formal psychometric testing. However, only 20% of patients with abnormalities have functionally significant deficits. Most of those with significant intellectual impairment have advanced disease and severe global dysfunction, but significant dementia occasionally occurs early in the disease. The most common findings are impaired memory, abstract reasoning, problem solving, and verbal fluency (Rao et al. 1984). The characteristic abnormality of memory is not with storage as much as with retrieval of recently learned material. There are ongoing studies (see LaRocca 1990) designed to evaluate the potential of cognitive rehabilitation for patients with limited impairments. It cannot be overemphasized that depression is common in MS and depressive symptoms may be mistaken for cognitive impairment (pseudodementia), even though a direct association between depression and cognitive impairment has not been demonstrated. The therapeutic importance of this distinction is obvious.

Fatigue. Most MS patients complain of fatigue, and many find this among the most disabling of symptoms (Freal et al. 1984). Descriptions variably include a "washed out," "exhausted," or "lacking in energy" sensation. It is usually most prominent in the mid- to late afternoon and is worsened by physical exercise and high ambient temperature and humidity. Rest, but not necessarily sleep, is usually restorative. The pathophysiological basis for MS-related fatigue is unknown, but conduction failure through partially demyelinated regions is suspected. Because many depressed patients complain of fatigue and because depression is frequent in MS, depression is a major differential diagnosis.

Some historical features distinguish MS-related fatigue from fatigue associated with depression. Patients with depression usually awaken in the morning feeling tired, whereas most patients with MS-related fatigue are at their best at this time. Although patients may describe considerable frustration with this symptom, the typical vegetative signs of depression are notably lacking. For example, patients with MS-related fatigue want to pursue their activities but cannot because of the fatigue, a situation much different from that of depressed individuals. Finally, fatigue can be a side effect of many medications used to treat other symptoms of MS.

Other symptoms. There are a variety of other symptoms that occasionally complicate the course of MS. Epilepsy occurs in about 5% of patients, a figure substantially higher than the prevalence of epilepsy in the general population. The many varieties of paroxysmal attacks such as the so-called tonic seizure (in which, for example, one limb suddenly and briefly assumes a dystonic posture) is uncommon but very characteristic of MS (Matthews 1975). Other paroxysmal attacks include paroxysmal dysarthria and ataxia, paroxysmal diplopia, and paroxysmal itching (Yamamoto et al. 1981). All of these share common characteristics, notably short duration (usually measured in seconds) and a tendency to occur many times daily. These phenomena are thought to reflect lateral transmission of nervous impulses across adjacent demyelinated tracts of the CNS (ephaptic transmission) (Matthews 1975).

Occasionally, MS patients will be found to have a Horner's syndrome. Many with advanced disease will have autonomic dysregulation of the cutaneous blood flow to the distal extremities, giving rise to a dusky erythema and dryness of the skin. There is an association between posterior uveitis and MS, usually characterized as perivenous sheathing as seen on funduscopy. Whether anterior uveitis occurs in MS is not settled. Finally, there are several references to peripheral nerve involvement in MS (e.g, Pollock et al. 1977). Some of these examples may represent a different disease, characterized by autoimmunity against shared antigenic components of peripheral and CNS myelin (overlap syndrome). It should be emphasized that a patient with prominent peripheral nerve abnormalities is unlikely to have MS or will, at least, be found to have another cause for the neuropathy.

Secondary Symptoms

The secondary problems are those that arise as a direct result of the neurological disturbances. They are a source of much morbidity in MS. More importantly, these problems are largely preventable if their occurrence is anticipated in patients at risk. Preventing secondary symptoms is probably the single most important role of health care providers who treat MS patients. Secondary problems include urinary tract infection (discussed above), fibrous contracture of muscles and ankylosis of joints, pressure sores, and aspiration pneumonia.

Fibrous contractures. Unremitting spasticity can lead to irreversible shortening of muscles which, especially in the lower limbs, can severely compromise patient positioning in a wheelchair or in bed. Once fibrous contractures have occurred, the only way to correct the resultant positioning problem is by tenotomy of the involved muscles. Moreover, fibrous contractures can lead to ankylosis of adjacent joints, further complicating management. Sometimes the extent of these complications may be difficult to appreciate because of coincidental spasticity, and it is occasionally necessary to examine the affected limbs under anesthesia, which relieves spasticity, so that the precise mechanism of severely altered posture can be determined. It is important that individuals with severely altered posture, especially those who have flexion deformities of the lower limbs, be considered for surgical correction. Otherwise, such individuals may develop pressure sores because of the inability to be properly positioned.

Pressure sores.   Pressure sores are primarily the consequence of sustained pressure of the tissues under bony prominences. In addition to postural abnormalities, alterations of the mental status, significant sensory impairment, and urinary incontinence accelerate their development. Without proper care, superficial skin lesions can quickly develop into deep ulcerations, which may extend, by sinus tracts, into adjacent joints or bones. Superficial sores can be managed conservatively, with the primary approach being prevention of further pressure until entirely healed. Deeper sores frequently require surgical management, which usually results in prolonged hospitalization.

Aspiration pneumonia.   Dysphagia is uncommon in MS and tends to be associated with advanced disease. Although incompletely studied in MS, it appears that the most common primary symptoms predisposing to dysphagia are pseudobulbar palsy and cerebellar disturbances affecting the oral-pharyngeal phase of swallowing. Many patients will have significant dysarthria as well. It is important that patients with dysphagia be thoroughly evaluated because aspiration pneumonia is a potentially life-threatening complication. Frequently, it is necessary to have the patient evaluated by a speech pathologist with experience in dysphagia. When the mechanism of dysphagia or the significance of the patient's complaints is not clear, performing a modified barium swallow with video fluoroscopy may help resolve the issue. Treatment for dysphagia may include restricting the diet to those foods and consistencies that the patient can safely swallow; however, some patients will require alternatives to oral intake, such as percutaneous gastrostomy.

Tertiary Symptoms

The tertiary symptoms include psychosocial and vocational problems that complicate the lives of many MS patients. Because it is unpredictable, MS is a disease that tends to cause considerable stress (LaRocca et al. 1987). The ability of MS patients to cope with this stress depends on the adequacy of their premorbid coping strategies and their internal and external support systems. External sources of support include relationships with family and friends, occupational affiliations, and medical interventions. Attitudes toward health and societal role, as well as preexisting stress-reducing strategies, constitute some of the internal support mechanisms. Patients with deficient or defective support systems lose their ability to adapt socially and psychologically as the impact of disease mounts. One of the many roles of the health care provider is to identify individuals with inadequate or failing coping strategies and provide them with the necessary assistance to reestablish control. Individual and family counseling and vocational rehabilitation, as well as referral to support groups such as the local chapters of the National Multiple Sclerosis Society, are ways that the health care provider can favorably influence outcome.

PROGNOSIS

Establishing a prognosis for an individual with MS is, at best, a tenuous exercise. Of course, it is extremely important to determine the prognosis so that patients and their families can prepare for the medical, social, and vocational problems that the disease may precipitate. MS is a disease whose course ranges from primarily benign, with as few as one or two neurological episodes of insignificant functional importance, to totally devastating, with total incapacity within months of onset. Further, it is by no means uncommon that a previously benign course suddenly becomes progressive with steadily increasing disability.

Despite these limitations, there are two broad general categories of MS: exacerbating-remitting and progressive (Kraft et al. 1977). The exacerbating-remitting type is characterized by episodes of clear-cut worsening that are not always associated with neurological signs on examination but are followed by total or near total resolution, usually within several weeks. In the progressive type, disability gradually mounts, and remissions, if any, are clearly incomplete.

Many neurologists familiar with the clinical course of MS would agree that there exists a group of patients with relapsing and remitting symptoms that are wholly sensory in nature and include episodes of dysesthesias, numbness, or visual loss. This characterizes the so-called benign or sensory MS, which, as the name suggests, is the most mild form of the disease and is not associated with disability. For many of these patients, their disease is merely an inconvenience, at least regarding the physical manifestations, and tends to have the most favorable long-term prognosis. Others with the exacerbating-remitting form have motor manifestations such as weakness, ataxia, or diplopia. It should be emphasized that patients with the exacerbating-remitting form of MS do not manifest significant disability even after many years of illness.

As its name suggests, the progressive type of MS is the most serious. Progressive MS can be divided further into a relapsing-progressive form and a chronic progressive form. Relapsing-progressive MS is characterized by clearly defined exacerbations but, as distinguished from exacerbating-remitting disease, recovery following the episodes is clearly incomplete. Over the years, disability gradually mounts. Patients with chronic progressive MS infrequently, if ever, have clear-cut exacerbations. Their course is characterized by a slow but steady progression of neurological impairment. Their history and physical examination usually suggest a myelopathic picture. Before the advent of newer diagnostic tests such as MRI, evoked potentials (EPs), and improved cerebrospinal fluid (CSF) analysis, these patients were the most difficult to diagnose because of the lack of evidence of dissemination of lesions on physical examination.

Although it is not possible to reliably determine the eventual outcome of an individual patient, some features of the history and findings on physical examination can help (Kurtzke et al. 1977). For example, frequent exacerbations, especially during the early phases of the illness, tend to be associated with a worse outcome than infrequent exacerbations. In those patients with relapsing-remitting disease, the average exacerbation frequency is about one episode every 2 years. When exacerbations are gradual in onset (i.e., evolving over weeks or months rather than days or a week or so), outcome is less favorable. Findings on physical examination indicating a poor prognosis are the early onset of persistent weakness or cerebellar dysfunction. As the foregoing would suggest, patients who have only sensory symptoms, including symptoms referable to the optic nerves, tend to have a favorable outcome.

Probably the single most important prognosticating factor is the Extended Disability Status Scale of Kurtzke (1983b). This is part of the Minimal Record of Disability for MS (Haber and LaRocca 1985) and is an ordinal scale that attempts to assign an estimate of disability based on findings on physical examination. The scale is heavily weighted in favor of gait abnormalities and is a good general reflection of global impairment. Several studies (Slater et al. 1984) have demonstrated that interrater reliability is high, and, when completed by persons familiar with it, use of this instrument over a period of years can give a general sense of the type of disease and the prognosis for a given patient. Thus this scale is important not only to assist in the selection of patients for experimental protocols for possible disease-modifying agents, but also for the purposes of vocational counseling.

DIAGNOSIS

Despite the advent of newer laboratory and radiological techniques, there is no specific diagnostic test, short of brain biopsy, for MS. The diagnosis of MS thus remains a clinical one, relying on the ability to demonstrate the existence of white matter lesions of the CNS that are disseminated in time and space. However, with judicious use of modern technological advances, the diagnosis can be reasonably secured.

The manifestations of MS vary remarkably from individual to individual because pathology can occur at almost any level of the CNS. There is, however, a definite predilection for certain structures, including the periventricular cerebral white matter, optic nerves, brain stem, cerebellum, and cervical spinal cord, resulting in the characteristic signs and symptoms.

It is worth emphasizing that no single finding is diagnostic of MS. Rather, it is the constellation of signs and symptoms, their historical development, and the results of various tests that provide the basis for diagnosis. Consequently, several attempts have been made over the years to use clinical and laboratory data to formulate the criteria from which a diagnosis of MS can be reasonably established. These schemes were originally developed to maintain consistency when admitting patients to therapeutic trials.

The Schumacher criteria (Schumacher et al. 1965) were concerned solely with identifying patients with clinically definite MS. These criteria continue to remain as valuable now as they were then for the diagnosis of MS. They can be summarized as follows:

1. Objective abnormalities on neurological examination that are attributable to CNS dysfunction. No symptom alone, no matter how typical, can be diagnostic of MS.
2. Evidence on clinical examination or by history of two or more separate white matter lesions. Involvement of more than one structure that can be explained by a single lesion is not acceptable.
3. Signs and symptoms must predominantly reflect white matter involvement, such as the optic nerves, long motor (corticospinal) and sensory (posterior column) tracts, brain stem, and cerebellum. Evidence of lower motor neuron dysfunction may occur, but must be minimal.
4. The course of illness must follow one of two patterns: either two or more episodes of neurological dysfunction separated by 24 hours or a slow, stepwise progression of signs and symptoms over a period of at least 6 months. The time limits attempt to exclude other neurological illnesses.
5. No better explanation for the patient's illness can be found. This "escape clause" admits that no set of criteria, no matter how thoughtfully designed, can substitute for the judgment of the careful and experienced clinician.

Many patients present with sufficient evidence on clinical grounds to support a diagnosis of MS. In the patient whose history suggests MS, but who does not have objective findings on examination to indicate two or more discrete CNS lesions (plaques), additional laboratory studies may be necessary to confirm the existence of clinically silent plaques. The tests most often used in the evaluation of MS are MRI, EP, and CSF analyses. Additionally, various expert urological procedures (e.g., cystometries) may be performed to assess symptoms suggestive of neurogenic bladder.

Diagnostic Tests

MRI. Because of its sensitivity in visualizing plaques of MS, MRI has become the single-most important advance in diagnosis. Characteristically, cerebral MRI reveals white matter plaques (seen as abnormally bright areas on T2-weighted images) in a periventricular distribution; similar changes may be found in the brain stem, cerebellum, and, less often, the spinal cord. A typical MRI pattern (Figure 1–1), although not specific for MS, can be found in over 85% of patients with clinically definite MS (Lukes et al. 1983; Robertson et al. 1987; Young et al. 1981). The clinical significance of the number and distribution of lesions remains a

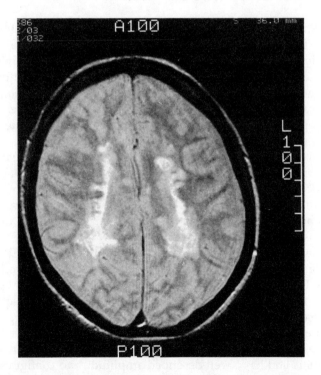

Figure 1–1. Cerebral magnetic resonance imaging (MRI) in a patient with clinically definite multiple sclerosis demonstrating increased periventricular white matter signals of T2-weighted imaging.

subject of much debate. There is little correlation with either neurological symptoms or degree of physical disability. However, it has been suggested that neuropsychiatric abnormalities in MS may be related to the extent of cortical white matter pathology seen on MRI (Rao et al. 1989). Other work has revealed that there are differences in the MRI pattern in patients with relapsing-remitting MS compared with that in patients with chronic progressive MS (Koopmans et al. 1989). Still, it is debatable whether MRI is useful in following and predicting disease course in MS. Thus, at present, MRI is best used as a diagnostic test to confirm dissemination of white matter lesions in a patient whose clinical presentation suggests MS. MRI abnormalities alone cannot be used to support the diagnosis of MS.

EP. EPs have been widely used for many years to demonstrate the presence of white matter lesions in MS (Chiappa 1980). Briefly, an EP is the electrical manifestation of the brain's response to an external stimulus. It is recorded as a computer-enhanced electric potential (wave) on the electroencephalogram. Clinical interpretation is based on the presence or absence of appropriate EP waves and their latencies (defined as the time elapsed from the onset of a stimulus to the wave peak).

Three types of EPs are used in the evaluation of MS: 1) pattern-shift visual, 2) brain stem auditory, and 3) somatosensory. These tests can provide reproducible and objective measures of function in their related sensory pathways. Their utility in MS rests on the ability to detect clinically asymptomatic lesions that are not disclosed on neurological examination.

The clinically interpreted visual evoked potential (VEP) is a single wave and is generated in the visual cortex of the occipital lobe. The preferred stimulus for investigation of the visual pathways is a shifting checkerboard pattern, in which the squares reverse color without change of total light output (Chiappa and Ropper 1982). The generated wave of interest (called the *P100*) appears approximately 100 milliseconds after the pattern-shift stimulus and has a well-described amplitude and configuration. VEPs with prolonged latencies and aberrant morphology are said to be abnormal. When MS is suspected, an abnormal VEP can demonstrate clinically silent lesions of the optic nerve. The inci-

dence of abnormal VEPs in MS has been reported to range from
50% to 96% (Halliday et al. 1973; Mastaglia et al. 1976), with an
average of 68% (Chiappa and Ropper 1982).

A brief auditory stimulus (click) to one ear produces sequen-
tial activation of the peripheral (auditory nerve) and central brain
stem auditory pathway in the pons and midbrain (the cochlear
and superior olivary nuclei, lateral lemniscus, and inferior col-
liculus), which generates a series of waves known as brain stem
auditory evoked potentials (BAEPs). Each of five waves (known
as *I, II, III, IV,* and *V*) represents a specific anatomic structure of
the auditory system, and fairly precise analysis of function can be
performed. Interpretation is based on measurements of the time
interval between waves, called *interpeak latencies* (Chiappa and
Ropper 1982). BAEPs are useful in demonstrating clinically silent
brain stem lesions in MS, but do so less frequently than VEPs.
Reported abnormalities have been shown in only 32%–64% of MS
patients (Chiappa et al. 1980; Kjaer 1980; Robinson and Rudge
1980). In patients without clinical evidence of brain stem lesions,
only one-fifth to one-half will have abnormal BAEPs (Chiappa
and Ropper 1982). Abnormalities found in MS include loss of
amplitude or absence of wave V, prolonged interwave latencies,
or both (Chiappa et al. 1980).

Somatosensory evoked potentials (SSEPs) are technically more
difficult to perform than VEPs or BAEPs. They are produced by
stimulation of peripheral nerves in the upper and lower extremities. Their reliability is thus dependent on an intact peripheral
nervous system (Eisen 1984). Conduction then proceeds through
the dorsal root ganglia, spinal cord (posterior columns), brain
stem (medial lemniscus), thalamus, and parietal cortex. When
performed correctly, SSEPs can demonstrate clinically silent lesions in the sensory pathway of the CNS. Clinical interpretation
is based on measurements of interwave latencies and central
conduction time. SSEPs with prolonged latencies and central
conduction times are considered to be abnormal. Side-to-side
differences in central conduction times, which usually vary by
less than 1.5 milliseconds, are especially sensitive indicators of
CNS disease (Eisen and Odusote 1980). Previous studies (Bartel
et al. 1983; Chiappa 1985) have found that approximately one-
half of patients with possible MS have abnormal SSEPs.

CSF. Although there is no specific CSF profile for MS, examination of the CSF can provide important clues in formulating a diagnosis. The most helpful CSF parameters are leukocyte count, total protein concentration, and immunoglobulin (IgG).

The total white blood cell count is normal (less than 5 cells/ mm^3) in 66% of patients with clinically definite MS; it is less than 20 cells/mm^3 in 99.7% of patients. Pleocytosis greater than 50 cells/mm^3 is rare and should suggest an alternative diagnosis (Tourtellotte 1970). The significance of these cells is uncertain, as there seems to be no consistent correlation between the degree of pleocytosis and disease activity.

The CSF concentration of total protein is normal (less than 54 mg/dl) in 77% of patients with clinically definite MS and less than 110 mg/dl in 99.7% of patients. Levels greater than 110 mg/dl are uncommon and should alert the clinician to the possibility of an alternative diagnosis (Tourtellotte 1970). The significance of the presence of myelin breakdown products, particularly myelin basic protein, in MS is controversial. CSF myelin basic protein may be elevated in 50%–90% of patients within 2 weeks before or after an MS exacerbation (Cohen et al. 1980; Whitaker et al. 1980). CSF myelin basic protein abnormalities are also seen in patients with strokes, head injury, and various CNS infections.

It has been well established that synthesis of IgG occurs at multifocal sites of inflammation in the CNS in MS. The proximity of MS lesions to the ventricular system permits entrance of intrinsically produced IgG to the CSF. Quantitative and qualitative analysis of CSF IgG yields abnormalities in almost all patients with clinically definite MS (Tourtellotte and Ma 1978). The rate of intra-blood-brain barrier synthesis of IgG is elevated in 88%–92% of patients with clinically definite MS (Link and Tibbling 1977; Tourtellotte 1970); this causes an increase in both the absolute and relative (compared with serum) CSF IgG concentration. (The relative IgG level in CSF can be calculated and is known as the *IgG index.*) Fractionation of IgG by CSF electrophoresis detects pathological oligoclonal bands in 97% of patients with clinically definite MS. Abnormal intra-blood-brain barrier IgG synthesis and/or oligoclonal IgG bands have been seen in 99% of patients (Tourtellotte et al. 1983).

New Diagnostic Criteria

The original clinical criteria for MS developed by Schumacher have been modified to take advantage of laboratory and radiological tests used in clinical neurology (Poser et al. 1983). Again, the classification is designed primarily for use in research protocols; it neither supplants the Schumacher criteria nor replaces the judgment of the careful and competent clinician.

In the new scheme (Table 1–1), an attack of MS is defined as the occurrence of a symptom or symptoms of neurological dysfunction, with or without objective confirmation, lasting more than 24 hours; historical information can be used if reliable and typical for MS. Attacks must involve different parts of the CNS and be separated by at least 1 month. Clinical evidence of a lesion provides signs of neurological dysfunction demonstrable by neurological examination. These signs are acceptable as evidence, even if no longer present, provided that they were previously

Table 1–1. New diagnostic criteria for multiple sclerosis

Category	Attacks	Clinical evidence		Paraclinical evidence	CSF OB/IgG
Clinically definite multiple sclerosis (CDMS)					
CDMS A1	2	2			
CDMS A2	2	1	and	1	
Laboratory-supported definite multiple sclerosis (LSDMS)					
LSDMS B1	2	1	or	1	+
LSDMS B2	1	2			+
LSDMS B3	1	1	and	1	+
Clinically probable multiple sclerosis (CPMS)					
CPMS C1	2	1			
CPMS C2	1	2			
CPMS C3	1	1	and	1	
Laboratory-supported probable multiple sclerosis (LSPMS)					
LSPMS D1	2				+

Note. OB/IgG = oligoclonal bands or increased immunoglobulins.
Source. Adapted from Poser et al. 1984.

elicited by a competent examiner. Paraclinical evidence is the demonstration of a lesion of the CNS by means of various tests and procedures (e.g., MRI and EP) that has not produced signs of neurological dysfunction but that may or may not have produced symptoms in the past. Laboratory support refers to the presence of oligoclonal bands or increased production of IgG in the CSF (CSF OB/IgG).

A diagnosis of clinically definite MS requires a history of two attacks. Evidence of two separate lesions of the CNS must then be provided by clinical and paraclinical testing. A diagnosis of laboratory-supported definite MS requires two attacks, either clinical or paraclinical evidence of one lesion, and the presence of CSF OB/IgG. Clinically probable MS is defined as two attacks with clinical evidence of one lesion or one attack with clinical or paraclinical evidence of two separate lesions.

DIFFERENTIAL DIAGNOSIS

The variable signs and symptoms of MS, both in their presentation and evolution, are commonly seen in many other diseases of the nervous system. The list of illnesses that can be confused with MS covers a fairly extensive area of clinical neurology and would be impossible to cover within the limitations of this chapter. In general, they can be categorized as 1) multifocal CNS diseases, 2) systematic CNS diseases, and 3) CNS diseases caused by single lesions.

Multifocal CNS Diseases

Multifocal CNS diseases include connective tissue diseases, vasculitis, sarcoidosis, chronic infections of the CNS, and other demyelinating diseases. These illnesses are often relapsing and remitting in nature, and each can produce findings on clinical examination, MRI, EP, and CSF that are seen in MS.

Systemic lupus erythematosus should be considered when there are signs of gray matter involvement (e.g., seizures and hemiparesis) and neuropsychiatric disturbances (e.g., psychosis and organic confusional states). Detection of antinuclear antibodies in the serum is useful in diagnosing systemic lupus erythematosus. Sjögren's syndrome (SS), associated with the sicca complex of dry eyes and dry mouth, as well as arthritis, can also produce disseminated CNS symptoms. Specific antibodies (SS-A and SS-B) can be found in patients with SS; their relationship to neurological disease is not known. Polyarteritis nodosa (systemic vasculitis) is usually accompanied by findings of systemic disease (e.g., anemia, weight loss, fever, leukocytosis, and increased erythrocyte sedimentation rate) and peripheral neuropathy. Granulomatous cerebral vasculitis is limited to the CNS without systemic manifestations. Neurological complications occur in 5% of patients with sarcoidosis; presence of multiple cranial palsies, hypothalamic dysfunction, elevated CSF protein, and hypercalcemia should raise the possibility of sarcoidosis. Behcet's syndrome can also produce multifocal CNS disease but is associated with recurrent uveitis and oral and genital ulcers; its etiology is unknown.

Chronic infections of the CNS that might be confused with MS include neurosyphilis and Lyme disease. Neurosyphilis is usually associated with pupillary abnormalities. Lyme disease, which is caused by the spirochete *Borrelia burgdorferi,* can also mimic MS and must be considered when there is a history of skin rash (erythema chronicum migrans), arthralgias, and meningeal symptoms; history of a tick bite may not always be elicited. Evidence of infection can be found using serological studies of serum and CSF.

Other demyelinating diseases that can be confused with MS include acute disseminated encephalomyelitis, adrenoleukodystrophy, and progressive multifocal leukodystrophy. Acute disseminated encephalomyelitis is a monophasic illness that is usually preceded by viral infection or vaccination and cannot be differentiated from the first episode of MS. Approximately 20% of patients with acute disseminated encephalomyelitis eventually develop MS. Adrenoleukodystrophy is an X-linked recessive disorder of males and is associated with adrenal insufficiency and elevated serum long-chain fatty acids. Adrenoleukodystrophy commonly presents with signs of peripheral nerve involvement. Progressive multifocal leukodystrophy is typically seen in patients who are immunocompromised, such as those with acquired immunodeficiency syndrome [AIDS] and those with lymphoma.

Systematic CNS Diseases

Diseases that are confined to specific systems within the CNS usually present with a symmetric, slowly progressive picture of neurological dysfunction. Many can be confused with MS. Progressive myelopathy as seen in the spinal form of MS can be seen in several other diseases of the spinal cord, which need to be differentiated from MS, including primary lateral sclerosis, tropical spastic paraparesis, and subacute combined degeneration.

Primary lateral sclerosis is a variant of motor neuron disease in which there is primarily slowly progressive degeneration of the pyramidal tracts of the spinal cord; bladder and sensory symptoms are rare. Spinal MRI may show atrophy of the cord.

Tropical spastic paraparesis is associated with chronic infection with human T-cell lymphotrophic virus type I (HTLV-I). Spastic paraparesis, mild sensory deficits in the lower extremities (usually diminished vibration and proprioception), and bladder dysfunction commonly occur. HTLV-I myelopathy is endemic to several tropical regions, including the Caribbean, Japan, and the Seychelle Islands. The diagnosis must be considered in patients native to these areas. Although the pathogenesis of the disorder has yet to be firmly elucidated, venereal and blood-borne transmission of HTLV-I is suspected. Diagnosis can be made by detecting antibodies to the virus in serum and CSF (Vernant et al. 1987).

Subacute combined degeneration is a consequence of vitamin B_{12} deficiency and is almost always associated with signs of peripheral neuropathy and macrocytic anemia.

The purely cerebellar form of MS must be differentiated from the hereditary group of spinocerebellar ataxias and paraneoplastic cerebellar degeneration. In spinocerebellar ataxia, MRI commonly demonstrates atrophy of the cerebellum and associated tracts in the brain stem. Paraneoplastic cerebellar degeneration is a subacute cerebellar disorder that progresses over weeks to months and is most often associated with Hodgkin's lymphoma, oat-cell carcinoma of the lung, and ovarian cancer (N. E. Anderson et al. 1988). Search for occult neoplasm should be performed in any patient with a pancerebellar syndrome of unknown etiology.

CNS Diseases Caused by Single Lesions

Localized disease of the nervous system can sometimes be confused with MS. Although usually associated with progressive neurological signs and symptoms, short "remissions" may occur, suggesting a diagnosis of MS. Conditions in this category include brain stem gliomas, cerebellopontine angle masses, deformities of the base of the skull (e.g., Arnold-Chiari malformation), foramen magnum tumors, and cerebral lymphoma, all of which can present with typical signs of MS. Vascular malformations of the brain stem and spinal cord may also present with intermittent symptoms. In addition, cervical spondylosis, tumors of the spinal cord and spinal roots (e.g., meningioma and neurofibroma), and syringomyelia may resemble MS in their early stages. MRI is extremely valuable in establishing the correct diagnosis.

When considering a diagnosis of MS the clinician must rely on both clinical and laboratory data, keeping in mind that no specific finding can in itself secure the diagnosis. Certain features of an illness do, however, argue against MS:

1. *Absence of optic nerve involvement.* Involvement of the optic nerves is extremely common in MS. In fact, VEP is one of the best tests for corroborating a second lesion when the diagnosis cannot be confirmed on clinical grounds. Because more than 75% of patients with definite MS have at least one abnormal VEP, a completely normal result should raise the possibility of an alternative diagnosis.
2. *Absence of oculomotor abnormalities.* These are very common in MS and are manifested variably.
3. *Absence of corticospinal tract signs.* A large percentage of patients with MS will have at least one Babinski response at some time during their course. This is not surprising as involvement of the pyramidal tract approaches 100% at autopsy in all reported studies.
4. *Absence of sensory dysfunction.* Sensory abnormalities in the lower extremities are nearly universal in MS.
5. *Absence of sphincteric impairment.* Bladder, bowel, and sexual complaints are characteristic of MS. Urinary symptoms are found in 75% of patients; constipation is even more frequent.

6. *Evidence for localized CNS disease.* Without evidence for dissemination of lesions, a diagnosis of MS must always be considered suspect. This is the most common reason to doubt a diagnosis of MS.

7. *Atypical signs and symptoms.* Aphasia, movement disorders, peripheral neuropathy, and isolated dementia are so unusual that their occurrence should immediately raise suspicion. In addition, moderate-to-severe motor disturbances without significant sensory or bladder impairment should lead the clinician to consider alternative diagnoses.

8. *Absence of a clinical remission, especially in a young patient.* The majority of patients who have progressive disease actually exhibit a relapsing and progressive course. Only 10%–15% of all patients have a clearly chronic progressive course without clear exacerbations; most are above the age of 50. A young patient with a slowly progressive course must be investigated to rule out tumor or degenerative disease.

9. *Normal or atypical MRI.* A typical MRI pattern is seen in more than 85% of cases of clinically definite MS. Overreading of images can lead to misdiagnosis if the clinical picture does not support a diagnosis of MS.

10. *Absence of CSF abnormalities or atypical CSF findings.* A majority of patients with clinically definite MS will have either oligoclonal bands or increased intrathecal IgG synthesis. Cell counts above 50 cells/mm^3 or a total protein above 110 mg/dl are so rare that they should immediately suggest another disease.

11. *"Tropical" MS.* One should recall the unequal geographic distribution of MS when making the diagnosis of MS in patients who have migrated from these areas after adolescence.

12. *Evidence of systemic illness.* Neurological manifestations of many disorders may be confused with MS. One must be cautious in making a diagnosis of MS in patients with other illnesses that may affect the nervous system.

In summary, despite strict adherence to the accepted diagnostic criteria for MS, it is possible to make errors because of its varied manifestations and lack of a specific diagnostic test. Diagnosis is based on a myriad of clinical and laboratory data; dependence on a single finding is not warranted. There still remains no substitute for a careful history, thorough examination, and sound clinical judgment.

REFERENCES

Anderson DW, Ellenberg JH, Leventhal CM, et al: Revised estimate of the prevalence of multiple sclerosis in the United States. Ann Neurol 31:333–336, 1992

Anderson NE, Rosenblum MK, Posner JB: Paraneoplastic cerebellar degeneration: clinical-immunologic correlations. Ann Neurol 24:559–567, 1988

Barrett M: Sexuality and Multiple Sclerosis. Toronto, Ontario, Multiple Sclerosis Society of Canada, 1977

Bartel DR, Markand ON, Kolar OJ: The diagnosis and classification of multiple sclerosis: evoked responses and spinal fluid electrophoresis. Neurology 33:611–617, 1983

Baum HM, Rothschild BB: The incidence and prevalence of reported multiple sclerosis. Ann Neurol 10:420–428, 1981

Beall SS, Concannon P, Charmley P, et al: The germline repertoire of T cell receptor beta-chain genes in patients with chronic progressive multiple sclerosis. J Neuroimmunol 21:59–66, 1989

Blaivas JG: Management of bladder dysfunction in multiple sclerosis. Neurology 30:12–18, 1979

Blaivas JG, Sinha HP, Zayed AAH, et al: Detrusor external sphincter dyssynergia. J Urol 125:542–544, 1981a

Blaivas JG, Sinha HP, Zayed AAH, et al: Detrusor external sphincter dyssynergia. J Urol 125:545–548, 1981b

Blaivas JG, Holland NJ, Giesser BG, et al: Multiple sclerosis bladder: studies and care. Ann N Y Acad Sci 436:326–345, 1984

Chiappa KH: Pattern-shift visual, brainstem auditory, and short-latency somatosensory evoked potentials in multiple sclerosis. Neurology 30 (7, part 2):110–123, 1980

Chiappa KH: Pattern-shift visual, brainstem auditory, and short-latency somatosensory evoked potentials in multiple sclerosis. Ann N Y Acad Sci 436:315–328, 1985

Chiappa KH, Ropper AH: Evoked potentials in clinical medicine. N Engl J Med 306:1140–1150, 1205–1211, 1982

Chiappa KH, Harrison JL, Brooks EB, et al: Brainstem auditory evoked responses in 200 patients with multiple sclerosis. Ann Neurol 7:135–143, 1980

Clifford DB, Trotter JL: Pain in multiple sclerosis. Arch Neurol 41:1270–1272, 1984

Cohen SR, Brooks BR, Herndon RM, et al: A diagnostic index of active demyelination: myelin basic protein in cerebrospinal fluid. Ann Neurol 8:25–31, 1980

Daugherty WT, Lederman RJ, Nodar RH, et al: Hearing loss in multiple sclerosis. Arch Neurol 40:33–35, 1983

Ebers GC, Bulman DE, Sadovnick AD, et al: A population based study of multiple sclerosis in twins. N Engl J Med 315:1638–1642, 1986

Eisen A: Use of the somatosensory evoked potential in multiple sclerosis, in The Diagnosis of Multiple Sclerosis. Edited by Poser CM, Paty DW, Scheinberg L, et al. New York, Thieme-Stratton, 1984, pp 131–139

Eisen A, Odusote K: Central and peripheral conduction times in multiple sclerosis. Electroencephalogr Clin Neurophysiol 48:253–265, 1980

Elian M, Dean G: Multiple sclerosis among the United Kingdom-born children of immigrants from the West Indies. J Neurol Neurosurg Psychiatry 50:327–332, 1987

Freal JE, Kraft GH, Coryell SK: Symptomatic fatigue in multiple sclerosis. Arch Phys Med Rehabil 65:135–138, 1984

Gilbert JJ, Sadler M: Unsuspected multiple sclerosis. Arch Neurol 40:533–536, 1983

Glick ME, Meshkinpoor H, Haldeman S: Colonic dysfunction in multiple sclerosis. Gastroenterology 83:1002–1007, 1982

Haber A, LaRocca N: Minimal Record of Disability in Multiple Sclerosis. New York, National Multiple Sclerosis Society, 1985

Hafler DA, Weiner HL: MS: a CNS and systemic autoimmune disease. Immunol Today 10:104–107, 1989

Halliday AM, McDonald WI, Mushin J: Visual evoked response in the diagnosis of multiple sclerosis. BMJ 4:661–664, 1973

Inman RP: Disability indices, the economic costs of illness, and social insurance: the case of multiple sclerosis. Acta Neurol Scand Suppl 70:46–55, 1984

Kalb RC, LaRocca NG, Kaplan SR: Sexuality, in Multiple Sclerosis: A Guide for Patients and Their Families, 2nd Edition. Edited by Scheinberg LC, Holland NJ. New York, Raven, 1987, pp 177–196

Kjaer M: Variations of brain stem auditory evoked potentials correlated to duration and activity of multiple sclerosis. Acta Neurol Scand 61:157–166, 1980

Koopmans RA, Li DKB, Grochowski E, et al: Benign versus chronic-progressive multiple sclerosis: magnetic resonance features. Ann Neurol 25:74–81, 1989

Kraft GH, Freal JE, Coryell JK: Multiple sclerosis: early prognostic guidelines. Journal of Chronic Disease. 30:819–830, 1977

Kurtzke JF: Geography in multiple sclerosis. J Neurol 215:1–26, 1977

Kurtzke JF: Epidemiology of MS, in Multiple Sclerosis. Edited by Hallpike JF, Adams CWM, Tourtellotte WW. Baltimore, MD, Williams & Wilkins, 1983a, pp 49–95

Kurtzke JF: Rating neurologic impairment in multiple sclerosis: an expanded disability status scale (EDSS). Neurology 33:1422–1427, 1983b

Kurtzke JF, Beebe GW, Nagler B, et al: Studies in the natural history of multiple sclerosis, VIII: early prognostic features of the later course of the illness. Journal of Chronic Disease 30:819–830, 1977

Kurtzke JF, Beebe GW, Norman JE: Epidemiology of multiple sclerosis in US veterans, I: race, sex, and geographic distribution. Neurology 29:1228–1235, 1979

LaRocca NG: A rehabilitation perspective, in Multiple Sclerosis: A Neuropsychological Perspective. Edited by Rao S. New York, Oxford University Press, 1990

LaRocca NG, Kalb RC, Kaplan SR: Psychological issues, in Multiple Sclerosis: A Guide for Patients and Their Families, 2nd Edition. Edited by Scheinberg LC, Holland NJ. New York, Raven, 1987, pp 197–213

Lassmann H: Comparative Neuropathology of Chronic Experimental Allergic Encephalomyelitis and Multiple Sclerosis. New York, Springer-Verlag, 1983

Levine JS: Bowel dysfunction in multiple sclerosis, in Interdisciplinary Rehabilitation of Multiple Sclerosis and Neuromuscular Disorders. Edited by Maloney FP, Burks JS, Ringel SP. Philadelphia, PA, JB Lippincott, 1985, pp 62–64

Link H, Tibbling G: Principles of albumin and IgG analyses in neurological disorders, I: establishment of reference values. Scand J Clin Lab Invest 37:397–401, 1977

Lukes SA, Crooks LE, Aminoff MJ, et al: Nuclear magnetic resonance imaging in multiple sclerosis. Ann Neurol 13:592–601, 1983

Mastaglia FL, Black JL, Collins DWK: Visual and spinal evoked potentials in the diagnosis of multiple sclerosis. British Medical Journal 2:732, 1976

Matthews WB: Paroxysmal symptoms in multiple sclerosis. J Neurol Neurosurg Psychiatry 38:617–623, 1975

Peyser JM, Edwards KR, Poser CM, et al: Cognitive function in patients with multiple sclerosis. Arch Neurol 37:577–579, 1980

Phadke JG, Best PV: Atypical and clinically silent multiple sclerosis: a report of 12 cases discovered unexpectedly at necropsy. J Neurol Neurosurg Psychiatry 46:414–420, 1983

Pollock M, Calder C, Allpress S: Peripheral nerve abnormality in multiple sclerosis. Ann Neurol 2:41–48, 1977

Poser CM, Paty DW, Scheinberg L, et al: New diagnostic criteria for multiple sclerosis: guidelines for research protocols. Ann Neurol 13:227–231, 1983

Poser CM, Paty DW, Scheinberg L, et al: The Diagnosis of Multiple Sclerosis. Edited by Poser CM, Paty DW, Scheinberg L, et al. New York, Thieme-Stratton, 1984, p 227

Rao SM, Hammeke TA, McQuillen MP, et al: Memory disturbance in chronic progressive multiple sclerosis. Arch Neurol 41:625–631, 1984

Rao SM, Leo GJ, Haughton VM, et al: Correlation of magnetic resonance imaging with neuropsychological testing in multiple sclerosis. Neurology 39:161–166, 1989

Robertson WD, Li DKB, Mayo JR, et al: Assessment of multiple sclerosis lesions by magnetic resonance imaging. J Can Assoc Radiol 38:177–182, 1987

Robinson K, Rudge P: The use of the auditory evoked response in the diagnosis of multiple sclerosis. J Neurol Sci 45:235–244, 1980

Sadovnick AD, Baird PA: The familial nature of multiple sclerosis: age-corrected empiric recurrence risks for children and siblings of patients. Neurology 38:990–991, 1988

Schumacher GA, Beebe G, Kibler RF, et al: Problems of experimental trials of therapy in multiple sclerosis: report by the panel on the evaluation of experimental trials of therapy in multiple sclerosis. Ann N Y Acad Sci 122:552–568, 1965

Slater R, LaRocca N, Scheinberg L: Development and testing of a Minimal Record of Disability in Multiple Sclerosis (in Multiple Sclerosis: Experimental and Clinical Aspects. Edited by Scheinberg L, Raine C). Ann N Y Acad Sci 436:453–468, 1984

Tourtellotte WW: Cerebrospinal fluid in multiple sclerosis, in Handbook of Clinical Neurology. Edited by Vinken PJ, Bruyn BW. Amsterdam, North Holland Publishing, 1970, p 324

Tourtellotte WW, Ma BI: Multiple sclerosis: the blood-brain-barrier and the measure of de novo central nervous system IgG synthesis. Neurology 28:76–83, 1978

Tourtellotte WW, Shapshak P, Staugaitis SM, et al: Do all clinical definite multiple sclerosis patients have evidence of intra-blood-brain-barrier synthesis (abstract)? Neurology 33 (suppl 2):123, 1983

Traugott U, Reinherz EL, Raine CS: Multiple sclerosis: distribution of T cells, T cell subset and Ia positive macrophages in lesions of different ages. J Neuroimmunol 4:201–221, 1983

Vernant JC, Maurs L, Gesain A, et al: Endemic tropical spastic paraparesis associated with human T-lymphotrophic virus type 1: a clinical and seroepidemiological study of 25 cases. Ann Neurol 21:123–131, 1987

Visscher BR, Detels R, Coulson AH, et al: Latitude, migration, and the prevalence of multiple sclerosis. Am J Epidemiol 106:470–475, 1977

Whitaker JN, Lisak RP, Bashir RM, et al: Immunoreactive myelin basic protein in the cerebrospinal fluid in neurologic disorders. Ann Neurol 7:58–64, 1980

Wynn DR, Rodriguez M, O'Fallon WM, et al: A reappraisal of the epidemiology of multiple sclerosis in Olmstead County, Minnesota. Neurology 40:780–785, 1990

Yamamoto M, Yabuki SK, Hayabara T, et al: Paroxysmal itching in multiple sclerosis: a report of three cases. J Neurol Neurosurg Psychiatry 44:19–22, 1981

Young JR, Hall AS, Pallis CA, et al: Nuclear magnetic resonance imaging of the brain in multiple sclerosis. Lancet 2:1063–1066, 1981

Chapter 2

Depression and Affective Disorders in Multiple Sclerosis

Sarah L. Minden, M.D., Randolph B. Schiffer, M.D.

T he mood disturbances associated with multiple sclerosis (MS) have been apparent to clinicians for many years. Charcot (1879) wrote that "it is not rare to see them give way to foolish laughter for no cause, and sometimes, on the contrary, melt into tears without reason. Nor is it rare, amid the state of mental depression, to find psychic disorders arise which assume one or other of the classic forms of mental alienation" (p. 160). Cottrell and Wilson (1926) insisted "that no single symptom of the neurological series (nystagmus, tremor, scanning speech, paraesthesiae, spasticity, amaurosis, etc.), occurs with anything like the same frequency in an unselected century of cases of the disease, and that the cardinal symptoms are not neurological, in its limited sense, but belong to the emotional, affective, and visceral spheres, and are constituted by: 1 Change in mood; 2 Change in bodily feeling; 3 Change in emotional expression and control" (pp. 16–17).

Nevertheless, it is only fairly recently that researchers have undertaken systematic studies of depression and other affective disturbances in MS (for a review, see Minden and Schiffer 1990). Similarly, clinicians now are paying closer attention to depressive symptoms reported by their patients and recommending psychiatric consultation and treatment (Minden et al. 1987a). In this chapter, we describe the psychological and social difficulties

This chapter is partially based on a previously published article (Minden SL, Schiffer RB: "Affective Disorders in Multiple Sclerosis: Review and Recommendations for Clinical Research." *Archives of Neurology* 47:98–104, 1990). Some sections of this chapter were presented at the annual meeting of the American Neuropsychiatric Association, Captiva Island, Florida, January 1990, and at the annual meeting of the American Psychiatric Association, New York, New York, May 1990.

experienced by people with MS; outline the present knowledge about the nature, etiology, and treatment of mood disorders in MS patients; and propose directions for future research.

BACKGROUND

The epidemiology, phenomenology, and pathophysiology of MS are discussed in detail in Chapter 1. We briefly review them here in the context of affective and cognitive disorders.

MS is the most common disabling neurological disease among young adults. The National Multiple Sclerosis Society estimates that there are 250,000 to 350,000 cases of MS in the United States (Anderson et al. 1992), with more than 10,000 new cases each year (Baum and Rothschild 1981; S. Reingold, personal communication, August 1992). Women are affected almost twice as often as men, with symptoms typically beginning when patients are in their twenties or thirties. The time between onset and diagnosis may be quite long—on average about 4 years (Gorman et al. 1984; Scheinberg et al. 1984)—primarily because initial symptoms may be mild and transient and because there is no specific diagnostic laboratory test. Such patients may experience considerable distress during this long period of uncertainty. There may be many doctor visits, multiple tests, and hospitalizations that contribute to anxiety, discouragement, and misunderstanding between patients and their physicians and family members. Errors in diagnosis are not rare, and a psychiatric diagnosis is frequently given rather than a neurological one.

In New Zealand, for example, Skegg et al. (1988) found that 16% of 91 MS patients were referred for psychiatric treatment during the time between the onset of their symptoms and the final diagnosis. The neurological disorder was missed entirely in more than half of these patients, regardless of typical MS symptoms. The diagnoses most often given were conversion reaction and hysterical personality disorder.

In MS, the myelin sheaths that insulate the nerve fibers are destroyed; although axons remain intact, nerve conduction is impaired. It is generally believed that a viral infection in childhood sensitizes the immune system to myelin antigens (Raine 1990). The acute lesion is an inflammatory one, that either resolves or progresses to scarring and demyelinated plaques. There is evidence to suggest that this process is a continuous one and that new lesions may develop up to 10 times more often than patients experience exacerbation of their symptoms (Willoughby and Paty 1990). Magnetic resonance imaging (MRI) and autopsy reports indicate that lesions may exist without symptoms and that symptoms may be present without observable lesions (Willoughby and Paty 1990). Plaques are most often found in the white matter around the lateral ventricles, although they can occur anywhere in the central nervous system (CNS). As a result of this diffuse and sporadic demyelination, patients vary enormously in the nature and severity of their symptoms and in the overall course and outcome of their illness.

At present, it is not possible to predict which individual patients will become disabled, although 50% of MS patients eventually will need ambulatory assistance (Biometry and Field Studies Branch, Intramural Research Program, National Institute of Neurological and Communicative Disorders and Stroke 1984). Of MS patients, 20% have a benign form of the disease, 25% have recurrent exacerbations with mild disability, 40% have a relapsing-progressive form of the illness with moderate-to-severe disability, and 15% have a progressive course with significant loss of function (Scheinberg and Holland 1987). Unpredictability is a major feature of MS and contributes to patients' difficulties in adjusting to their illness: patients' lives are disrupted by both unexpected exacerbations and day-to-day fluctuations in symptoms. Because MS usually begins when patients are just establishing their careers and families, the disability, unpredictability, and uncertain outcome produce profound effects on all aspects of life.

Although difficulty with walking, incoordination, and unusual sensations are the most well-known symptoms of MS, visual, speech, and cognitive problems may also be present. Further, incontinence contributes to social isolation, and fatigue—affecting nearly 90% of patients (Freal et al. 1984)—may be a major impediment to work. The impact of an individual's symptoms depends on his or her life situation. Even mild weakness, tremor, or cerebellar symptoms may end a dancer's career, whereas a teacher's livelihood will be threatened by dysarthria and memory impairment. MS cannot, at this time, be cured, and symptomatic treatments bring only limited relief.

There are significant economic, social, and interpersonal consequences of MS. By 10 to 15 years after onset, more than 60% of MS patients are unemployed (Colville 1983; Kornblith et al. 1986; Kraft et al. 1986; LaRocca et al. 1985; Minden et al. 1987b; Mitchell 1981; Poser et al. 1981), and people with MS who do continue working generally work fewer hours or take on less taxing jobs. A 1976 survey found that, on average, the cost of MS to patients and their families was $15,000 per year in health care and lost income; this represented roughly a 44% loss of income per household (Biometry and Field Studies Branch, Intramural Research Program, National Institute of Neurological and Communicative Disorders and Stroke 1984; Inman 1984). Two studies (Braham et al. 1975; Power 1985) have described significant marital discord in 53%–72% of couples in which one person had MS, and two studies (Arnaud 1959; Power 1985) have reported high levels of dysphoria, anxiety, and behavioral and interpersonal problems among children who had a parent with MS. Furthermore, 40% of MS patients spend most of the day alone, and 50% lack adequate family or outside social support (Braham et al. 1975; Colville 1983; Harper et al. 1986).

DEPRESSION

Whether it is a response to the physical, social, and economic problems described above or the result of brain disease, depression is common among MS patients. Table 2–1 shows that recent estimates of the current prevalence of depression range from 14% to 57% and that estimates of lifetime prevalence range from about 37% to 54%. This variation may be due to differences in sample characteristics and diagnostic techniques or may reflect the variability inherent in MS. Minden and colleagues (Minden et al. 1987a; see also, Weissman and Myers 1978) found that, in their sample of patients, the rate of major depression before the onset of neurological symptoms was not significantly different from the lifetime rate of major depression for 26–45 year olds in a community population. After the onset of MS symptoms, however, the rate of major depression was found to be significantly

Table 2–1. Prevalence of depression in patients with multiple sclerosis (MS)

Study	Sample size[a]	Duration of MS in years[b]	Severity of MS[c]	Method	Prevalence (%) Current	Since onset of MS	Lifetime
Cottrell and Wilson 1926	100 (0)	0–5 (51) 6–9 (29) 10–19 (16) 20+ (4)	—	Int	10	10	
Sugar and Nadell 1943	28 (0)	0–5 (33) 6–9 (17) 10–19 (35) 20+ (15)	Subjects in chronic care hospital	Int	18	25	
Braceland and Giffin 1950	75 (0)	—	—	Int	20		
Pratt 1951	100 (100)[d]	—	Mild (43) Moderate (39) Severe (18)	Int		45	
Surridge 1969	108 (39)[e]	0–5 (15) 6–10 (54) 11–15 (23) 16–25 (8)	Minimal (23) Mild (7) Moderate (38) Severe (32)	Int	27		
Kahana et al. 1971	295 (0)	mean 17.3	?	Chart review	6		

(*continued*)

Table 2–1. Prevalence of depression in patients with multiple sclerosis (MS) *(continued)*

Study	Sample size[a]	Duration of MS in years[b]	Severity of MS[c]	Method	Prevalence (%) Current	Prevalence (%) Since onset of MS	Prevalence (%) Lifetime
Whitlock and Siskind 1980	30 (30)[d]	0–4 (20) 5–9 (53) 10–14 (13) 15+ (13)	Minimal (47) Mild (40) Moderate (10) Severe (3)	Int BDI	57	53	
Schiffer et al. 1983	30 (15)[f]	—	— ?	SADS, DSM-III, BDI		37	
Joffe et al. 1987	100 (0)	—	DSS mean 5.3±1.9	SADS, RDC BDI, HDRS	14	25	42
Minden et al. 1987a	50 (0)	mean 11.3±7.7	DSS mean 4.2±2.1	SADS, RDC BDI, HDRS	16	54	54

Note. Int = interview; BDI = Beck Depression Inventory (Beck et al. 1961); SADS = Schedule for Affective Disorders and Schizophrenia (Endicott and Spitzer 1979); DSM-III = Diagnostic and Statistical Manual of Mental Disorders, 3rd Edition (American Psychiatric Association 1980); RDC = Research Diagnostic Criteria (Endicott and Spitzer 1979); DSS = Kurtzke Disability Status Scale (Kurtzke 1961); HDRS = Hamilton Depression Rating Scale (Hamilton 1960)
[a]N control subjects presented in parentheses
[b]Percentage of patients presented in parentheses
[c]Percentage of patients presented iin parentheses
[d]Neurological patients
[e]Muscular dystrophy patients
[f]Healthy adults

higher than an age-adjusted rate for the community sample.

Symptoms of depression in MS patients tend to be moderately severe (Joffe et al. 1987; Minden et al. 1987a; Whitlock and Siskind 1980), most typically anger, irritability, worry, and discouragement (Table 2–2) (Minden et al. 1987a). Suicide rates are unknown, although a study by Kahana et al. (1971) in Israel found that 3% of 295 MS patients died by suicide between 1960 and 1966. Whitlock and Siskind (1980) found 1 completed suicide, 1 attempted suicide, and 13 patients with suicidal ideas in a sample of 30 MS patients. Among the 50 patients interviewed by Minden et al. (S. L. Minden, J. Orav, P. Reich, unpublished data, January 1984), 5 had moderately serious suicidal preoccupations at the time of interview, and 6 had previously made a total of 10 suicide attempts. Two chapters of the National Multiple Sclerosis Society that surveyed 136,631 persons found 21 completed suicides (B. Waksman, personal communication, November 1989). Finally, a study (Whitlock 1982) of 1,052 suicides in Great Britain found

Table 2–2. Depressive symptoms reported by 50 patients with multiple sclerosis

Symptom[a]	*n* patients reporting symptom	%
Dysphoria	32	64
Anger	32	64
Irritability	28	56
Worry	24	48
Discouragement	21	42
Bodily concern	19	38
Poor concentration	19	38
Self-reproach	19	38
Social withdrawal	18	36
Negative view of self	18	36
Anxiety	17	34
Loss of interest	14	28

[a]Schedule for Affective Disorders and Schizophrenia (Endicott and Spitzer 1979)
Source. From Minden SL, Schiffer RB: "Mood Disorders in Multiple Sclerosis." *Neuropsychiatry, Neuropsychology, and Behavioral Neurology* 4:62–77, 1991. Used with permission.

CNS disease in 69: MS in 6; cerebrovascular accidents in 18; epilepsy in 19; cerebrovascular disease and other degenerative conditions in 11; head injury or cerebral tumors in 8; and other, nonspecified conditions in 7.

Investigators have tried to determine whether depression in MS patients results from a psychological reaction to serious illness or from demyelination of limbic structures. Indirect evidence that demyelination plays a central role lies in two observations: 1) depressive episodes are more frequent in samples of MS patients than in the general population (Minden et al. 1987a), groups of control subjects (Baldwin 1952), patients with other medical (Minden et al. 1987a) and neurological (Whitlock and Siskind 1980) illnesses, and patients with disabling disorders that do not affect the CNS, such as spinal cord injury (Dalos et al. 1983; Rabins et al. 1986) or amyotrophic lateral sclerosis (Schiffer and Babigian 1984), and 2) MS patients whose disease primarily involves the cerebrum appear to have higher rates of depression than do patients with mainly spinal cord lesions (Rabins et al. 1986; Schiffer et al. 1983). Some (e.g., Goodstein and Ferrell 1977; Joffe et al. 1987; Matthews 1979; Whitlock and Siskind 1980) have argued that when depressive episodes precede the onset of other MS symptoms they are an early sign of demyelination. Because the age at onset is similar for recurrent unipolar depression and MS, it is possible, of course, that these MS patients have two distinct disorders.

Other findings are even more ambiguous and could suggest either an association between depression and demyelination or a psychodynamic interpretation. For example, although it seems clear that depressive symptoms are more common when patients are in exacerbation than when they are in remission (Cleeland et al. 1970; Dalos et al. 1983), it is not known whether they are a manifestation of disease activity or an emotional response to the concomitant loss of function, fatigue, and malaise.

Some investigators (e.g., McIvor et al. 1984; Whitlock and Siskind 1980) have found a relationship between depression and severity of disability, whereas others (e.g., Minden et al. 1987a; Rabins et al. 1986) have not. Sample differences may explain these divergent results. Studies reporting an association between disability and depression may contain more patients who are acutely disabled because of an exacerbation (when depression is more common) than do studies in which the patients are disabled primarily because of the chronic progression of their illness. Indeed, research has shown that longer duration of symptoms (which correlates with severity of disability) is associated with more successful adjustment, presumably because of the opportunity to adapt over time (Brooks and Matson 1982). This highlights how necessary it is for investigators to describe their patients' current disease activity status.

There is general agreement, however, that depression is not directly related to the type of disability (e.g., motor, bowel and bladder, or visual) (Minden et al. 1987a; Rabins et al. 1986), the type of MS (e.g., exacerbating-remitting or progressive) (Minden et al. 1987a), the duration of symptoms (McIvor et al. 1984; Minden et al. 1987a; Rabins et al. 1986; Whitlock and Siskind 1980), or cognitive function (Minden et al. 1990).

It is unlikely that major depression in MS is due to inheritance of a primary affective disorder as both Minden et al. (1987a) and Joffe et al. (1987) found that the rate of depression in first-degree relatives was the same for MS patients with major depression and MS patients without major depression. By contrast, some evidence points to a possible shared genetic vulnerability between MS and bipolar disorder. Both Joffe et al. (1987) and Schiffer et al. (1986) found significantly higher than expected rates of bipolar illness among MS patients, and Schiffer et al. (1988) reported on familial clustering of MS and bipolar disorder. Further, Schiffer et al. (1988) also described possibly nonrandom inheritance of certain major histocompatibility class II markers among patients with both MS and bipolar disorder (see also, Cazzullo et al. 1983).

Minden et al. (1988) found that of 50 MS patients, 9 became hypomanic or manic in response to treatment with adrenocorticotropic hormone (ACTH) and prednisone. These patients had family histories of affective disorder or alcoholism and personal histories of previous depressive episodes. Several case reports (e.g., Garfield 1985; Kellner et al. 1984; Kemp et al. 1977; Mapelli and Ramelli 1981; Matthews 1979; Peselow et al. 1981; Solomon 1978) have also documented the coexistence of mania and MS.

New technologies, such as MRI, may help clarify whether mood disorders result from CNS changes due to disease. Honer et al. (1987), comparing MRI scans of eight MS patients with psychiatric disorders (six of whom had bipolar or unipolar depression) to eight matched nonpsychiatric MS control subjects, found no difference in the total volume of brain affected, but a greater proportion of plaques were within the temporal lobes of the patients with psychiatric disorders. Reischies et al. (1988) reported a significant correlation between depressed mood and periventricular plaques observed on MRI.

Treatment of Depression

Little is known about effective treatment for depression in MS. In a double-blind, placebo-controlled study of desipramine in 28 MS patients with major depression, Schiffer and Wineman (1990) found significantly greater improvement in those treated with desipramine, although almost 40% of patients developed side effects with doses equal to or greater than 125 mg/day. Improvement in depression has been demonstrated in controlled studies of insight-oriented group psychotherapy and cognitive-behavior group therapy (Crawford and McIvor 1985; Larcombe and Wilson 1984). Although there have not been any studies of treatment for bipolar disorder in MS patients, two case reports (Kellner et al. 1984; Kemp et al. 1977) suggest that lithium carbonate effectively controls mania; in a third study (Peselow et al. 1981) a manic MS patient had a variable response.

Along with the lack of research on treatment of depression in MS, clinicians may not be treating depressed MS patients as effectively as possible. Although 38 of the 50 patients in the study by Minden et al. (1987a) had a major, minor, or intermittent depression in the preceding year, only 22 received some type of treatment (Table 2–3).

Assessment of Depression

Most of the studies on depression and MS have significant methodological problems. Typically, patients come from teaching hospitals and clinics rather than from the general population of MS patients; in many studies, patients have not been randomly selected. The most severely disabled patients are usually excluded, and only a few studies contain control subjects. It is not clear, however, what population would be the most appropriate comparison group (spinal cord injury patients, used in some studies, have comparable disabilities, but not other key features of MS [e.g., unpredictable and fluctuating symptoms]).

Most, but not all, recent studies have moved beyond subjective diagnoses by administering structured interviews (e.g., the Schedule for Affective Disorders and Schizophrenia [Endicott and Spitzer 1979] and the Hamilton Depression Rating Scale [Hamilton 1960]) and formal diagnostic criteria (e.g., the Research Diagnostic Criteria [Endicott and Spitzer 1979] and DSM-III-R [American Psychiatric Association 1987]). Self-report instruments such as the Beck Depression Inventory (Beck et al. 1961) or the General Health Questionnaire (Goldberg and Hillier 1979) may be confounded by cognitive impairment, lack of motivation, and poor insight (Gottlieb et al. 1988).

Interviews have the advantage of providing data on past episodes and permitting diagnosis of psychiatric disorders rather than simply identifying clusters of symptoms. Because fatigue, slowed thinking, and poor concentration are present in both MS and depression, diagnostic interviews should be modified to exclude these symptoms from the criteria for diagnosis, and self-

Table 2–3.   Treatment of 38 multiple sclerosis patients with depression

Treatment[a]	Major depression[b] ($n = 17$)	Minor and intermittent depression[b] ($n = 21$)
Lithium	3	0
Tricyclic antidepressant	4	2
Anxiolytic	4	3
Neuroleptic	0	1
Mental health consultation	2	1
Treatment by a mental health professional for 2 weeks or more	4	8
Psychiatric hospitalization	1	0
No psychiatric treatment	5	11

[a]Patients may have had multiple treatments
[b]Research Diagnostic Criteria (Endicott and Spitzer 1979)
Source. From Minden SL, Schiffer RB: "Mood Disorders in Multiple Sclerosis." *Neuropsychiatry, Neuropsychology, and Behavioral Neurology* 4:62–77, 1991. Used with permission.

report instruments should be submitted to appropriate statistical analyses to determine whether somatic symptoms are biasing the results. Research interviewers should clarify for patients the difference between depressive psychomotor retardation and MS-related fatigue, between crying from sadness and pathological weeping, and between depressive loss of interest and physical inability to perform an activity (Minden et al. 1987a). It is preferable that investigators employ self-report questionnaires that are widely used to facilitate comparisons between studies.

EUPHORIA

"Euphoria" has often been used loosely to characterize almost any form of emotional disturbance in MS; unfortunately, it is still considered by some to be a hallmark of the disease. Euphoria should be distinguished from hypomania and mania. Euphoric MS patients do not exhibit hyperactivity, pressured speech, or racing thoughts; nor do they have transitory shifts in mood. Rather, they have a sustained "mental state of cheerfulness, happiness, [and] ease—expressed negatively by the absence of mental uneasiness, anxiety, tension, or dispeace" (Cottrell and Wilson 1926, p.8). Euphoric patients appear "serene and cheerful" (Cottrell and Wilson 1926). Even as they describe their severe physical disabilities, euphoric patients may also report feeling physically fit and healthy, and display "an optimism as to the future and the prospects of ultimate recovery which is out of place and incongruous" (Cottrell and Wilson 1926, p. 8).

Euphoria is neither a reversible mood nor a fluctuating emotional state. It represents a permanent change in personality and a new, persistent frame of mind and outlook. It is as if patients' attitudes and demeanors had become dissociated from their objective knowledge about themselves and their conditions. There is also a dissociation between their outward expression of emotion and their inner mood: the emotional responses expected from a severely disabled person are not observable, and, in some cases, the apparent lack of concern hides a significant depression (Sugar and Nadell 1943; Surridge 1969). There is no consensus on the prevalence of euphoria in MS. There is a large range in the rates reported in the literature (Table 2–4), from zero to 63%,

Table 2–4. Prevalence of euphoria in multiple sclerosis (MS)

Study	Sample size[a]	Duration of MS in years[b]		Severity of MS[c]		Method	Prevalence (%)
Cottrell and Wilson 1926	100 (0)	0–5 6–9 10–19 20+	(51) (29) (16) (4)	—		Interview	63
Langworthy et al. 1941	199 (0)	—		—		Chart review	13
Sugar and Nadell 1943	28 (0)	0–5 6–9 10–19 20+	(33) (17) (35) (25)	Subjects in chronic care hospital		Interview	54
Braceland and Giffin 1950	75 (0)	—		—		Interview	10
Pratt 1951	100 (100)[d]	—		Mild Moderate Severe	43 39 18	Interview	7

(continued)

Table 2–4. Prevalence of euphoria in multiple sclerosis (MS) *(continued)*

Study	Sample size[a]	Duration of MS in years[b]		Severity of MS[c]		Method	Prevalence (%)
Baldwin 1952	34 (34)[e]	0–5	(47)	Minimal	(20)	Interview	0
		6–10	(26)	Mild	(15)		
		11–15	(15)	Moderate	(30)		
		16–20	(9)	Severe	(35)		
		20+	(3)				
Surridge 1969	108 (39)[f]	0–5	(15)	Minimal	(23)	Interview	26
		6–10	(54)	Mild	(54)		
		11–15	(23)	Moderate	(38)		
		16–25	(8)	Severe	(32)		
Kahana et al. 1971	295 (0)	mean 17.3		—		Chart review	5
Rabins et al. 1986	87 (16)[g]	mean 8.6 ± 6.8		—		Neurologist rating	48

[a] N control subjects presented in parentheses
[b] Percentage of patients presented in parentheses
[c] Percentage of patients presented in parentheses
[d] Neurological patients
[e] Healthy women
[f] Muscular dystrophy patients
[g] Spinal cord injury patients

probably because there is no standardized definition of euphoria.

Euphoria in MS is not a psychological process, but a neurologically based emotional state (Cottrell and Wilson 1926; Kahana et al. 1971; Langworthy et al. 1941; Rabins et al. 1986; Sugar and Nadell 1943; Surridge 1969), the result of demyelination presumably of the frontal lobes, basal ganglia, and parts of the limbic system (Mur et al. 1966; O'Malley 1966; Salguero et al. 1969). It is related to severe disability, long duration of symptoms, the chronic progressive type of MS, enlarged ventricles on computed tomography (CT) scan, and cognitive impairment (Rabins et al. 1986; Surridge 1969). It is not associated with disease involving only the spinal cord or with depression (Rabins et al. 1986).

There is, at present, no treatment for euphoria, but neither families nor patients find it unpleasant. When family members are troubled by an MS patient's indifference, it is often useful to assure them that euphoria is not uncommon and is part of the disease process.

PATHOLOGICAL LAUGHING AND WEEPING

Pathological laughing and weeping is also a neurologically based condition, a syndrome of emotional dysregulation that does not involve the patient's subjective emotional state, but only the outward display of emotion. Although patients with pathological laughing and weeping report that they do not feel sad or depressed, they will burst into tears at the slightest provocation. Both euphoric and noneuphoric patients with MS may experience pathological laughing and weeping. Prevalence rates are unknown and highly variable (Table 2–5).

Although not thoroughly understood, pathological laughing and weeping most likely results from disconnection of diencephalic or brain stem centers from right hemisphere or frontal control. One retrospective study (Sackheim et al. 1982) found an association with damage to the right hemisphere in right-handed persons, but others (e.g., Langworthy and Hesser 1940) have suggested that bilateral damage is necessary. In stroke patients, this disorder has been associated with pontine brain stem lesions or lesions connecting the middle right cerebral hemispheres with the pons (Tatemichi et al. 1987; Yarnell 1987).

Table 2–5. Prevalence of pathological laughing and weeping in multiple sclerosis (MS)

Study	Sample size[a]	Duration of MS in years[b]		Severity of MS[c]		Method	Prevalence (%)
Cottrell and Wilson 1926	100 (0)	0–5 6–9 10–19 20+	(51) (29) (16) (4)	—		Interview	95
Langworthy et al. 1941	199 (0)	—		—		Chart review	7
Sugar and Nadell 1943	28 (0)	0–5 6–9 10–19 20+	(33) (17) (35) (15)	Subjects in chronic care hospital		Interview	79
Pratt 1951	100 (100)[d]	—		Mild Moderate Severe	(43) (39) (18)	Interview	51
Surridge 1969	108 (39)[e]	0–5 6–10 11–15 16–25	(15) (54) (23) (8)	Minimal Mild Moderate Severe	(23) (7) (38) (32)	Interview	5

[a]N control subjects presented in parentheses
[b]Percentage of patients presented in parentheses
[c]Percentage of patients presented in parentheses
[d]Neurological patients
[e]Muscular dystrophy patients

Pathological laughing and weeping may resolve with low doses (25–75 mg/day) of amitriptyline (Schiffer et al. 1985). Levodopa may also be useful (Udaka et al. 1984; Wolf et al. 1979).

FUTURE DIRECTIONS FOR RESEARCH

We have much more to learn about affective disorders in MS. Large population-based studies are needed to determine accurate prevalence and incidence rates and the natural history of the various mood disorders. Depressive disorders should be diagnosed on the basis of structured interviews and strict diagnostic criteria; objective scales for determining the presence and severity of euphoria and pathological laughing and weeping need to be developed. Rather than comparing MS patients with other populations, more careful study of MS patients themselves may demonstrate how those who develop mood disorders differ from those who do not.

Serial MRI scanning may help clarify the neuroanatomical structures involved and the relationship between changes in mood and disease activity. Investigation of neuroendocrine and immunological function in depressed MS patients and of the neurotransmitter systems involved in the response of pathological laughing and weeping to amitriptyline and levodopa may broaden our understanding of the neurochemistry of emotional regulation.

Family history studies followed by studies employing molecular genetic techniques may clarify the hypothesized genetic link between MS and bipolar illness. Finally, double-blind, placebo-controlled studies of medications and careful investigation of individual and group psychotherapies will enhance our ability to treat mood disorders in MS patients more effectively. Above all, the simplistic question that has guided investigators to this point—do mood disorders arise from organic brain disease or from psychological responses to illness?—should be reframed in the light of current understanding. There is considerable individual variation and a wide variety of predisposing factors involved in the mood disorders with MS.

REFERENCES

American Psychiatric Association: Diagnostic and Statistical Manual of Mental Disorders, 3rd Edition. Washington, DC, American Psychiatric Association, 1980

American Psychiatric Association: Diagnostic and Statistical Manual of Mental Disorders, 3rd Edition, Revised. Washington, DC, American Psychiatric Association, 1987

Anderson DW, Ellenberg JH, Leventhal CM, et al: Revised estimates of the prevalence of multiple sclerosis in the United States. Ann Neurol 31:333–336, 1992

Arnaud SH: Some psychological characteristics of children of multiple sclerotics. Psychosom Med 21:8–21, 1959

Baldwin MV: A clinico-experimental investigation into the psychologic aspects of multiple sclerosis. J Nerv Ment Dis 115:299–342, 1952

Baum HM, Rothschild BB: The incidence and prevalence of reported multiple sclerosis. Arch Neurol 10:420–428, 1981

Beck AT, Ward CH, Mendelson M, et al: An inventory for measuring depression. Arch Gen Psychiatry 4:561–571, 1961

Biometry and Field Studies Branch, Intramural Research Program, National Institute of Neurological and Communicative Disorders and Stroke: Multiple Sclerosis: A National Survey. Bethesda, MD, NIH Publication No. 84-2479, 1984

Braceland FJ, Giffin ME: The mental changes associated with multiple sclerosis: an interim report. Res Publ Assoc Res Nerv Ment Dis 28:450–455, 1950

Braham S, Houser HB, Cline A, et al: Evaluation of the social needs of nonhospitalized chronically ill persons, I: study of 47 patients with multiple sclerosis. Journal of Chronic Diseases 28:401–419, 1975

Brooks NA, Matson RR: Social-psychological adjustment to multiple sclerosis. Soc Sci Med 16:2129–2135, 1982

Cazzullo CL, Smeraldi E, Gasperini M, et al: Preliminary correlation between primary affective disorders and multiple sclerosis, in New Trends in Multiple Sclerosis Research. Edited by Cazzullo CL, Caputo D, Ghezzi A. Milan, Italy, Masson Italia Editori, 1983, pp 57–62

Charcot JM: Lectures on the diseases of the nervous system delivered at la Salpêtrière. Philadelphia, PA, Henry C Lea, 1879

Cleeland CS, Matthews CG, Hopper CL: MMPI profiles in exacerbation and remission of multiple sclerosis. Psychol Rep 27:373–374, 1970

Colville PL: Rehabilitation, in Multiple Sclerosis Pathology, Diagnosis, and Management. Edited by Halpike JF, Adams CWM, Tourtelotte WW. Baltimore, MD, Williams & Wilkins, 1983, pp 631–654

Cottrell SS, Wilson SAK: The affective symptomatology of disseminated sclerosis. Journal of Neurology and Psychopathology 7:1–30, 1926

Crawford JD, McIvor GP: Group psychotherapy: benefits in multiple sclerosis. Arch Phys Med Rehabil 66:810–813, 1985

Dalos NP, Rabins PV, Brooks BR, et al: Disease activity and emotional state in multiple sclerosis. Ann Neurol 13:573–583, 1983

Endicott J, Spitzer RL: Use of the Research Diagnostic Criteria and the Schedule for Affective Disorders and Schizophrenia to study affective disorders. Am J Psychiatry 136:52–56, 1979

Freal JF, Kraft GH, Coryell JD: Symptomatic fatigue in multiple sclerosis. Arch Phys Med Rehabil 65:135–138, 1984

Garfield DAS: Multiple sclerosis and affective disorders: two cases of mania with psychosis. Psychother Psychosom 44:22–33, 1985

Goldberg DP, Hillier VF: A scaled version of the General Health Questionnaire. Psychol Med 9:139–145, 1979

Goodstein RK, Ferrell RB: Multiple sclerosis—presenting as depressive illness. Diseases of the Nervous System 38:127–131, 1977

Gorman E, Rudd A, Ebers GC: Giving the diagnosis of multiple sclerosis, in The Diagnosis of Multiple Sclerosis. Edited by Poser CM, Paty DW, Scheinberg LC, et al. New York, Thieme-Stratton, 1984, pp 205–215

Gottlieb GL, Gur RE, Gur RC: Reliability of psychiatric scales in patients with dementia of the Alzheimer type. Am J Psychiatry 145:857–860, 1988

Hamilton M: A rating scale for depression. J Neurol Neurosurg Psychiatry 23:56–62, 1960

Harper AC, Harper DA, Chambers LW, et al: An epidemiological description of physical, social and psychological problems in multiple sclerosis. Journal of Chronic Diseases 39:305–310, 1986

Honer WG, Hurwitz T, Li DKB, et al: Temporal lobe involvement in multiple sclerosis patients with psychiatric disorders. Arch Neurol 44:187–190, 1987

Inman RP: Disability indices, the economic costs of illness, and social insurance: the case of multiple sclerosis. Acta Neurol Scand Suppl 101:46–55, 1984

Joffe RT, Lippert GP, Gray TA, et al: Mood disorder and multiple sclerosis. Arch Neurol 44:376–378, 1987

Kahana E, Leibowitz U, Alter M: Cerebral multiple sclerosis. Neurology 21:1179–1185, 1971

Kellner CH, Davenport Y, Post RM, et al: Rapidly cycling bipolar disorder and multiple sclerosis. Am J Psychiatry 141:112–113, 1984

Kemp K, Lion JR, Magram G: Lithium in the treatment of a manic patient with multiple sclerosis: a case report. Diseases of the Nervous System 38:210–211, 1977

Kornblith AB, LaRocca NTG, Baum HM: Employment in individuals with multiple sclerosis. Int J Rehab Res 9:155-165, 1986

Kraft GH, Freal JE, Coryell JK: Disability, disease duration, and rehabilitation service needs in multiple sclerosis: patient perspective. Arch Phys Med Rehabil 67:164–168, 1986

Kurtzke JF: On the evaluation of disability in multiple sclerosis. Neurology 11:686–694, 1961

Langworthy OR, Hesser FH: Syndrome of pseudobulbar palsy; an anatomic and physiologic analysis. Arch Intern Med 65:106–121, 1940

Langworthy OR, Kolb LC, Androp S: Disturbances of behavior in patients with disseminated sclerosis. Am J Psychiatry 98:243–249, 1941

Larcombe NA, Wilson PH: An evaluation of cognitive-behaviour therapy for depression in patients with multiple sclerosis. Br J Psychiatry 145:366–371, 1984

LaRocca N, Kalb R, Scheinberg L, et al: Factors associated with unemployment of patients with multiple sclerosis. Journal of Chronic Diseases 38:203–210, 1985

Mapelli G, Ramelli E: Manic syndrome associated with multiple sclerosis: secondary mania? Acta Psychiatr Belg 81:337–349, 1981

Matthews B: Multiple sclerosis presenting with acute remitting psychiatric symptoms. J Neurol Neurosurg Psychiatry 42:859–863, 1979

McIvor GP, Riklan M, Reznikoff M: Depression in multiple sclerosis as a function of length and severity of illness, age, remissions, and perceived social support. J Clin Psychology 40:1028–1033, 1984

Minden SL, Schiffer RB: Affective disorders in multiple sclerosis: review and recommendations for clinical research. Arch Neurol 47:98–104, 1990

Minden SL, Schiffer RB: Mood disorders in multiple sclerosis. Neuropsychiatry, Neuropsychology, and Behavioral Neurology 4:62–77, 1991

Minden SL, Orav J, Reich P: Depression in multiple sclerosis. Gen Hosp Psychiatry 9:426–434, 1987a

Minden SL, Orav J, Moes E, et al: Social adjustment in multiple sclerosis. Paper presented at the Symposium on Mental Disorders, Cognitive Deficits, and Their Treatment in Multiple Sclerosis, Odense, Denmark, November 1987b

Minden SL, Orav J, Schildkraut JJ: Hypomanic reactions to ACTH and prednisone treatment for multiple sclerosis. Neurology 38:1631–1634, 1988

Minden SL, Moes EJ, Orav J, et al: Memory impairment in multiple sclerosis. J Clin Exp Neuropsychol 12:566–586, 1990

Mitchell JN: Multiple sclerosis and the prospects for employment. J Soc Occup Med 31:134–138, 1981

Mur J, Kumpel G, Dostal S: An anergic phase of disseminated sclerosis. Confinia Neurologica 28:37–49, 1966

O'Malley PP: Severe mental symptoms in disseminated sclerosis: a neuro-pathological study. J Irish Med Assoc 58:115–127, 1966

Peselow ED, Fieve RR, Deutsch SI, et al: Coexistent manic symptoms and multiple sclerosis. Psychosomatics 22:824–825, 1981

Poser S, Bauer HG, Ritter G, et al: Rehabilitation for patients with multiple sclerosis. J Neurol 224:283–290, 1981

Power PW: Family coping behaviors in chronic illness: a rehabilitation perspective. Rehabil Lit 46:78–83, 1985

Pratt RTC: An investigation of the psychiatric aspects of disseminated sclerosis. J Neurol Neurosurg Psychiatry 14:326–335, 1951

Rabins PV, Brooks BR, O'Donnell P, et al: Structural brain correlates of emotional disorder in multiple sclerosis. Brain 109:585–597, 1986

Raine CS: Neuropathology, in Neurobehavioral Aspects of Multiple Sclerosis. Edited Rao SM. New York, Oxford University Press, 1990, pp 15–36

Reischies FM, Baum K, Brau H, et al: Cerebral magnetic resonance imaging findings in multiple sclerosis: relation to disturbance of affect, drive, and cognition. Arch Neurol 45:1114–1116, 1988

Sackheim HA, Greenberg MS, Weiman AL, et al: Hemispheric asymmetry in the expression of positive and negative emotions. Arch Neurol 39:210–218, 1982

Salguero LF, Itabashi HH, Gutierrez NB: Childhood multiple sclerosis with psychotic manifestations. J Neurol Neurosurg Psychiatry 32:572–579, 1969

Scheinberg LC, Holland NJ: MS: A Guide for Patients and Their Families, 2nd Edition. New York, Raven, 1987

Scheinberg LC, Kalb RC, LaRocca NG, et al: The doctor-patient relationship in multiple sclerosis, in The Diagnosis of Multiple Sclerosis. Edited by Poser CM, Paty DW, Scheinberg LC, et al. New York, Thieme-Stratton, 1984, pp 205–215

Schiffer RB, Babigian HM: Behavioral disorders in multiple sclerosis, temporal lobe epilepsy, and amyotrophic lateral sclerosis: an epidemiologic study. Arch Neurol 41:1067–1069, 1984

Schiffer RB, Wineman NM: Antidepressant pharmacotherapy of depression associated with multiple sclerosis. Am J Psychiatry 147:1493–1497, 1990

Schiffer RB, Caine ED, Bamford KA, et al: Depressive episodes in patients with multiple sclerosis. Am J Psychiatry 140:1498–1500, 1983

Schiffer RB, Herndon RM, Rudick RA: Treatment of pathologic laughing and weeping with amitriptyline. N Engl J Med 312:1480–1482, 1985

Schiffer RB, Wineman NM, Weitkamp LR: Association between bipolar affective disorder and multiple sclerosis. Am J Psychiatry 143:94–95, 1986

Schiffer RB, Weitkamp LR, Wineman NM, et al: Multiple sclerosis and affective disorders: family history, sex, and HLA-DR antigens. Arch Neurol 45:1345–1348, 1988

Skegg K, Corwin PA, Skegg DCG: How often is multiple sclerosis mistaken for a psychiatric disorder? Psychol Med 18:733–736, 1988

Solomon JG: Multiple sclerosis masquerading as lithium toxicity. J Nerv Ment Dis 166:663–665, 1978

Sugar C, Nadell R: Mental symptoms in multiple sclerosis. J Nerv Ment Dis 98:267–280, 1943

Surridge D: An investigation into some psychiatric aspects of multiple sclerosis. Br J Psychiatry 115:749–764, 1969

Tatemichi TK, Nichols FT, Mohr JP: Pathological crying: a pontine pseudobulbar syndrome (abstract). Ann Neurol 22:133, 1987

Udaka F, Yamao S, Nagata H, et al: Pathologic laughing and crying treated with levodopa. Arch Neurol 41:1095–1096, 1984

Weissman MM, Myers JK: Affective disorders in a U.S. urban community: the use of research diagnostic criteria in an epidemiological survey. Arch Gen Psychiatry 35:1304–1311, 1978

Whitlock FA: The neurology of affective disorder and suicide. Aust N Z J Psychiatry 16:1–12, 1982

Whitlock FA, Siskind MM: Depression as a major symptom of multiple sclerosis. J Neurol Neurosurg Psychiatry 43:861–865, 1980

Willoughby EW, Paty DW: Brain imaging in multiple sclerosis, in Neurobehavioral Aspects of Multiple Sclerosis. Edited by Rao SM. New York, Oxford University Press, 1990, pp 37–62

Wolf JK, Santana HB, Thorpy M: Treatment of "emotional incontinence" with levodopa (letter). Neurology (Minneapolis) 29:1435–1436, 1979

Yarnell PR: Pathological crying localization (abstract). Ann Neurol 22:133, 1987

Chapter 3

Cognitive and Neuroimaging Changes in Multiple Sclerosis

Stephen M. Rao, Ph.D.

I n his Salpêtrière lectures, Charcot (1877) viewed cognitive dysfunction as a hallmark symptom of patients with multiple sclerosis (MS). Specifically, he described his patients as having a "marked enfeeblement of the memory" with "conceptions [that are] formed slowly." With the recent application of neuropsychological testing methods, considerable progress has been achieved in understanding the cognitive symptoms that Charcot so astutely described. This chapter is divided into two sections. In the first section, I provide a comprehensive review of the scientific literature regarding cognitive dysfunction in MS. In the second section, I examine the clinicopathologic correlations between measures of cognitive dysfunction and neuroimaging techniques.

COGNITIVE DISTURBANCE IN MS

Recent neuropsychological studies have shown that cognitive dysfunction is a common occurrence in MS patients. Several recent reviews of this research area have appeared in the scientific literature (e.g., Peyser et al. 1990; Rao 1990a). In the following section, I briefly summarize the current understanding of 1) the prevalence of cognitive dysfunction in MS, 2) the most common patterns of dysfunction, 3) the relationship between cognitive dysfunction and physical disability and other illness variables, 4) the impact of cognitive dysfunction on employment and social functioning, 5) the relationship between affective disorders and

The research cited in this chapter was supported in part by a Research Career Development Award (K04 NS01055) and a Research Grant (RO1 NS22128) from the National Institute of Neurological Disorders and Stroke and Research Grants (RG2206-A-3, RG2028-A-2) from the National Multiple Sclerosis Society.

cognitive dysfunction, 6) methods for screening cognitive dysfunction, and 7) treatments of cognitive dysfunction.

Prevalence

Large-scale population studies that have assessed cognitive dysfunction using informal mental status examinations (e.g., Kurtzke et al. 1970) suggest that less than 5% percent of MS patients have cognitive dysfunction. In contrast, neuropsychological studies (e.g., Bertrando et al. 1983; De Smedt et al. 1984; Heaton et al. 1985; Lyon-Caen et al. 1986; Parsons et al. 1957; Peyser et al. 1980; Rao et al. 1984; Staples and Lincoln 1979; Truelle et al. 1987) indicate a prevalence rate between 54% and 65%. These neuropsychological studies may be criticized, however, for assessing a biased patient population: patients attending university-based medical centers. Such patients have greater physical disability and more active disease than the MS population in general (Nelson et al. 1988). In a recent study of 100 community-based MS patients, Rao et al. (1991b) obtained an overall prevalence estimate of 43%.

Patterns of Cognitive Dysfunction

In patients with MS who exhibit cognitive dysfunction, there is nonuniform decline in cognitive functions. Particular deficits are noted on measures of recent memory (Beatty and Gange 1977; Beatty et al. 1988, 1989; Caine et al. 1986; Carroll et al. 1984; Fischer 1988; Grant et al. 1984; Jambor 1969; Litvan et al. 1988a; Minden et al. 1990; Rao et al. 1984, 1989c, 1991b), conceptual and abstract reasoning (Beatty et al. 1989; Jambor 1969; Parsons et al. 1957; Rao and Hammeke 1984; Rao et al. 1987, 1991b; Vowels and Gates 1984), sustained attention (Litvan et al. 1988b; Rao et al. 1991b; van den Burg et al. 1987), information-processing speed (Litvan et al. 1988b; Rao et al. 1989a, 1991b), visuospatial skills (Rao et al. 1991b), and verbal fluency (Beatty et al. 1988; Caine et al. 1986; Rao et al. 1989c, 1991b; van den Burg et al. 1987). On recent and remote memory measures, MS patients' deficits appear to be the result of faulty retrieval as MS patients perform normally or near normally on recognition testing (Caine et al. 1986; Carroll et al. 1984; Rao et al. 1984, 1989c, 1991b; van den

Burg et al. 1987). On the other hand, immediate (i.e., span) memory (Heaton et al. 1985; Jambor 1969; Litvan et al. 1988a, 1988b; Rao et al. 1984, 1989c; Staples and Lincoln 1979), language functions (Jambor 1969; Rao et al. 1991b), and general intellectual functions (Rao 1986) appear to be relatively well preserved. This pattern of deficits is similar to that observed in other so-called subcortical dementias, such as Parkinson's disease, Huntington's disease, and progressive supranuclear palsy (Rao 1990c), and different from that seen in Alzheimer's disease, a cortical dementia producing intellectual decline due to amnesia, aphasia, and agnosia (Filley et al. 1989).

Relationship to Physical Disability and Other Illness Variables

Severity of cognitive dysfunction in MS patients is either not correlated or weakly correlated with physical disability (Marsh 1980; Peyser et al. 1980; Rao et al. 1984, 1991b; van den Burg et al. 1987), as measured by the Kurtzke Expanded Disability Status Scale (EDSS) (Kurtzke 1983). The EDSS is heavily influenced by the patient's ability to ambulate. As such, a lesion in the brain stem or spinal cord could produce severe physical disability, but have no effect on cognitive abilities. Conversely, patients with predominantly "cerebral" disease may have little problems with ambulation yet exhibit significant cognitive deterioration.

Neuropsychological studies have not found significant correlations between duration of illness and cognitive impairment (Ivnik 1978; Marsh 1980; Rao et al. 1984, 1991b). Some investigators have noted that cognitive dysfunction can appear early in the disease (Lyon-Caen et al. 1986; Young et al. 1976), sometimes before the establishment of the diagnosis (Callanan et al. 1989). All of these studies have relied on cross-sectional research designs. A controlled, prospective, long-term (3-year), longitudinal study of cognitive dysfunction in MS is currently under way at the Medical College of Wisconsin in Milwaukee.

A few studies (e.g., Heaton et al. 1985; Rao et al. 1987) have noted that patients with a chronic progressive course are more likely to experience cognitive dysfunction than are patients with a relapsing-remitting or stable course. This relationship was not found by others (e.g., Beatty et al. 1990; Rao et al. 1991a).

A significant number of MS patients experience mood disorders (Minden and Schiffer 1990), which are treated with psychoactive medications. Most neuropsychological studies have found that medications (Rao et al. 1989a, 1991b) and mood disorder (Jambor 1969; Lyon-Caen et al. 1986; Rao et al. 1991b) contribute little, if anything, to explain the cognitive problems of MS patients.

Impact on Employment and Social Functioning

Several investigators (Franklin et al. 1989; Marsh 1980; Staples and Lincoln 1979) have noted that MS patients are more impaired in activities of daily living than would be predicted on the basis of physical disability alone. In a recently completed study, Rao et al. (1991a) found that cognitively impaired MS patients were less likely to be employed, engaged in fewer social activities, and required greater personal assistance than did cognitively intact MS patients. In addition, cognitive impairment was associated with sexual dysfunction and significantly poorer performance on measures of activities of daily living (e.g., following recipes). These findings were particularly striking because the two groups did not differ in gender, age, education, premorbid occupational status, overall level of physical disability on the EDSS, or duration of illness.

Relationship Between Affective Disorders and Cognitive Dysfunction

The early literature on personality disturbance suggested that a significant percentage of MS patients were euphoric (Cottrell and Wilson 1926; Sugar and Nadell 1943). More recent studies (Joffe et al. 1987; Schiffer et al. 1986; Whitlock and Siskind 1980) have emphasized the high rate of depression, both unipolar and bipolar, among MS patients compared with the rate in the general population. Notwithstanding the methodological problems of measuring mood disturbance in this population (Minden and Schiffer 1990; Rao and Leo 1988), it would appear that affective disorders are common, although the precise causes (i.e., biological or psychological) are unknown.

A few studies have examined the relationship between cognitive dysfunction and mood disorder. Rabins et al. (1986) found that euphoric mood (rated by the investigators) was more common in patients with cognitive dysfunction. Rao et al. (1991a) had close relatives or friends rate the behavior of a large sample of MS patients using the Katz Adjustment Scale (Katz and Lyerly 1963). Cognitively impaired MS patients were more likely to be rated as more confused, less emotionally stable, more helpless, and more socially withdrawn than were cognitively intact MS patients. These differences did not appear to be related to patients' self-rating of depression on the Zung Self-Rating Depression Scale (Zung 1965). Therefore, it is very likely that cognitively impaired MS patients exhibit a personality change similar to that observed in patients with prefrontal lobe brain damage (Stuss and Benson 1984). This change is frequently characterized by apathy, lack of initiation, and increased irritability.

Screening for Cognitive Dysfunction

Given that approximately one-half of MS patients have cognitive dysfunction, it would be useful to have a screening instrument that could validly discriminate cognitively impaired from cognitively intact MS patients. Traditional screening instruments, such as the Mini-Mental State Exam (MMSE) (Folstein et al. 1975), have proven to be relatively insensitive to the cognitive deficits in MS (Beatty and Goodkin 1990; Rao et al. 1991b). Rao et al. (1991b) constructed a brief (20-minute) screening instrument by selecting the most sensitive measures in a 7-hour neuropsychological test battery (see also, Rao et al. 1989d). This brief battery yielded sensitivity and specificity values of 71% and 94%, respectively, in discriminating cognitively intact from impaired MS patients as defined by the longer battery. In contrast, the MMSE achieved acceptable specificity (98%), but unacceptable sensitivity (23%).

Treatment

Very little has been reported in the literature pertaining to the treatment of cognitive deficits in MS patients. Although considerable efforts have been expended to develop cognitive retraining programs for patients with stroke and closed head trauma (Ben-Yishay and Diller 1983), no studies have evaluated retraining procedures in MS. This is somewhat surprising, as MS is the most common, nontraumatic, neurological illness affecting young and middle-aged adults (Johnson et al. 1979) and, as noted above, MS-related cognitive dysfunction can have a devastating impact on employment and social functioning.

Leo and Rao (1988) reported a placebo-controlled, double-blind, cross-over study of *intravenous* physostigmine, an acetyl-cholinesterase inhibitor, as a treatment for memory loss in four MS patients. Patients receiving physostigmine had better scores on the Selective Reminding Test (SRT) (Buschke 1973), a measure of recent memory functioning, than while receiving placebo. As a follow-up to this study, Unverzagt et al. (1991) recently completed a double-blind, placebo-controlled, cross-over, long-term (1-month) study of oral physostigmine administered to 10 memory-impaired MS patients. As in the previous intravenous study, patients exhibited improvement on the SRT, but neither the patients nor their family members observed a change in everyday memory functioning.

NEUROIMAGING CHANGES IN MS

Autopsy studies (Adams 1977; Brownell and Hughes 1962; Powell and Lampert 1983) indicate that the cerebral hemispheres are commonly affected in MS patients. The most common lesions are observed in the white matter surrounding the lateral ventricles, although lesions may also be observed in the gray-white matter junction (Brownell and Hughes 1962). Ventricular dilatation is also frequently noted in the brains of MS patients, presumably due to thinning of the periventricular white matter (Brownell and Hughes 1962).

Recent advances in brain imaging (i.e., computed tomography [CT], magnetic resonance imaging [MRI], and positron-emission tomography [PET]) have made it possible to correlate MS-related brain changes with measures of cognitive test performance. Depending on the imaging modality, four indicators of cerebral pathology have been examined: 1) ventricular dilatation, 2) total lesion burden, 3) lesion location, and 4) regional changes in cerebral physiology. In this section, I summarize the clinicopathologic correlations obtained from examining each of these indices.

Ventricular Dilatation

Compared with MRI, the standard, unenhanced CT scan images have not been particularly useful in detecting cerebral lesions in MS (Haughton et al. 1979). However, age-inappropriate cerebral atrophy has been found in approximately 40% of MS patients on CT scan (Rao et al. 1985). Cerebral atrophy, therefore, may serve as an indirect, albeit late, marker of cerebral disease activity in MS. Three studies have correlated measures of cerebral atrophy with cognitive testing.

Brooks et al. (1984) administered the Wechsler Adult Intelligence Scale (WAIS) (Wechsler 1955), standardized reading tests, and CT scans to 12 MS patients. Eight patients exhibited cerebral atrophy on CT scan. Seven of these 8 patients exhibited cognitive dysfunction, whereas the 4 patients without atrophy showed no signs of cognitive decline.

Rabins et at. (1986) examined 37 MS patients with CT and the MMSE and performed ratings of "euphoric mood state." Their results indicated that patients with large ventricles were more likely to be impaired cognitively and to be rated as "euphoric." A significant correlation was observed between a linear measure of atrophy and MMSE scores ($r = .33$).

Rao et al. (1985) obtained subjective ratings of ventricular size from CT scans from 47 chronic progressive MS patients. The cognitive measures included the verbal subtests of the Wechsler Adult Intelligence Scale—Revised (WAIS-R) (Wechsler 1981), the Wechsler Memory Scale (Wechsler 1956), and two experimental measures of verbal and visuospatial learning and memory. CT scans were classified as having either no, mild, or moderate-to-severe cerebral atrophy. Nineteen patients (40%) were judged to have no ventricular enlargement, 19 (40%) had mildly enlarged ventricles, and 9 (20%) had moderate-to-severe ventricular dilatation. Statistically significant ($P < .05$) group differences were observed on the WAIS-R comprehension subtest and on 10 of 13 measures of learning and memory. In a later study, Rao (1990b) compared the correlations between cognitive performance and three CT atrophy measures: 1) blind subjective ratings, 2) linear measurements (Huckman et al. 1975), and 3) ventricular volume measures, computed as a ventricular-brain ratio (VBR). Significant, albeit weak, correlations ($r = .30$ to $.40$) were obtained for subjective ratings and VBR; linear measurements were poor indicators of cognitive test performance.

Total Lesion Burden

The introduction of MRI has emphasized the significant involvement of the cerebrum in MS patients. For every lesion observed on the unenhanced CT scan, approximately 20 lesions are observed on MRI scans (Jacobs et al. 1986; Lukes et al. 1983; Young et al. 1981). The shape, location, and distribution of lesions on MRI scans closely resemble those observed at autopsy (Willoughby and Paty 1990).

Six studies (Anzola et al. 1990; Baumhefner et al. 1990; Franklin et al. 1988; Huber et al. 1987; Medaer et al. 1987; Rao et al. 1989d) have correlated the extent of brain involvement on MRI with neuropsychological testing in patients with MS. Only two of these studies (Baumhefner et al. 1990; Rao et al. 1989d) used quantitative measures of lesion burden; the remainder used subjective ratings of disease burden.

Huber et al. (1987) obtained a weighted lesion score based on the number and size of lesions scored from the MRIs of 30 definite MS patients. Size of lesion was rated on a 5-point scale. A brief (30-minute) battery of neuropsychological tests, including the MMSE and measures of language, memory, apraxia, visuospatial ability, and depression (Zung Self-Rated Depression Scale), was administered. On the basis of this testing protocol, 9 patients (28%) were classified as "demented," 11 (34%) were moderately impaired, and 12 (38%) were minimally impaired. No significant group differences were observed on lesion scores, although the patients classified as "demented" had greater corpus callosum atrophy.

Medaer et al. (1987) administered neuropsychological testing (WAIS, Raven Progressive Matrices [Raven 1960], Rey Auditory Verbal Learning Test [Rey 1964], and an attentional task) to 33 definite MS patients. Patients were classified into 3 groups of 11 each on the basis of test performance: normal cognitive functions, "partial" impairment, and "serious" impairment. MRI scans were rated on a single 5-point scale based on the size and number of lesions and the degree of cerebral atrophy. Mean MRI ratings were significantly higher ($P < .05$) in the "partial" and "serious" patient groups compared with the cognitively intact group; no differences were observed between the two cognitively impaired groups on MRI ratings.

Franklin et al. (1988) recorded the number and size (using a 3-point scale) of lesions from 60 patients with chronic progressive MS. A weighted lesion score was computed based on the number and size of lesions; these scores were summed to obtain an overall brain lesion score. This score correlated significantly ($r = .35$) with a summary score derived from a brief (30- to 45-minute) cognitive screening battery. Anzola et al. (1990) divided 41 MS patients into two groups: 19 without and 22 with extensive periventricular demyelination. The latter group performed significantly worse on measures of verbal memory, nonverbal problem solving, and concept formation.

In the first study to use a quantitative index of total lesion area, Rao et al. (1989d) administered a 7-hour battery of neuropsychological tests, consisting of measures of verbal intelligence, memory, abstract and conceptual reasoning, attention and concentration, language, and visuospatial skills, to 53 definite or probable MS patients. Lesion areas were measured by tracing the outlines of lesions on the MRI scanner computer console; software routines computed the area (in cm^3) subtended by each tracing. A total lesion area (TLA) was computed by adding the measurements of lesion size. The investigators also recorded the quantitative measures of VBR and size of the corpus callosum (SCC). Stepwise multiple regression analyses indicated that TLA correlated strongly ($r = .40$ to $.54$) with measures of recent memory, abstract and conceptual reasoning, verbal fluency, and visuospatial reasoning. SCC correlated equally strongly with the measures of sustained attention and mental processing speed. VBR did not independently predict cognitive test performance.

Baumhefner et al. (1990) measured TLA and sustained attention, with the Symbol Digit Modalities Test (SDMT) (Smith 1973), in 62 MS patients. Performance on the SDMT correlated .49 for TLA derived from axial slices, and .52 for TLA measured from coronal slices.

It would appear that subjective ratings of lesion burden are poor predictors of cognitive test performance when compared with quantitative measures. Correlations with subjective ratings account for less than 10% of the shared variance with cognitive testing. In contrast, correlations with quantitative measures account for more than 25%–30% of the explained variance. Quantitative measures of lesion burden are also superior to measures of ventricular dilatation. These studies indicate that, although virtually all definite MS patients have abnormal MRI results (Lukes et al. 1983), the overall lesion burden is directly proportional to the amount of cognitive dysfunction.

Lesion Location

Several studies have suggested that focal areas of brain involvement in MS are associated with specific patterns of cognitive disruption. Brainin et al. (1988), for example, found that bilateral lesions in the hippocampal regions in 5 MS patients were associated with severe impairment on measures of recent memory, whereas patients with moderate ($n = 10$) or no memory problems ($n = 5$) had either unilateral or no hippocampal lesions.

Rao et al. (1989b) examined the hypothesis that MS patients with atrophy of the corpus callosum would demonstrate a reduction in interhemispheric information transfer. Previous studies (Jacobson et al. 1983; Rubens et al. 1985) had shown that patients with MS exhibit left-ear suppression to dichotically presented verbal stimuli. Rao et al. (1989b) were able to replicate these previous findings, but only for patients with significant corpus callosum atrophy. In addition, this effect could also be achieved for the visual modality using a tachistoscopic object-naming latency task; only patients with significant corpus callosum atrophy were slow at naming objects presented to their left visual field.

Regional Changes in Cerebral Physiology

Only one study has examined the possible relationship between degree of cognitive dysfunction and altered cerebral physiology as imaged by PET. Brooks et al. (1984) measured regional cerebral oxygen utilization, oxygen extraction, blood flow, and blood volume in 15 MS patients in remission. Patients were administered intelligence and reading tests; 13 patients also underwent CT scanning. Compared with a non-MS control group (n = 13), cerebral oxygen utilization and blood flow were found to be reduced in both the white and peripheral gray matter of the MS patients. This effect was most dramatic in patients with ventricular dilatation on CT scan and in patients with a significant drop in intelligence relative to a prediction of premorbid cognitive ability (i.e., based on reading test scores). They concluded that reduced blood flow in MS is diffuse and caused by a loss of cerebral brain tissue rather than by cerebral ischemia.

CONCLUSIONS

The past ten years have witnessed a substantial increase in our knowledge of cognitive disorders in MS. We now know that approximately 40%–45% of MS patients develop a subcortical dementia, characterized predominantly by forgetfulness, slowed mental processing, sustained attentional problems, and impaired conceptual reasoning. This dementia is unrelated to physical disability, affective disturbance, or medication usage, but is strongly related to the amount of cerebral brain involvement on MRI. The rate of progression of the dementia is not known, although several longitudinal studies are currently under way.

Cognitive dysfunction can have a significant impact on an MS patient's quality of life. Unfortunately, very little attention has been devoted to the treatment of these disorders. Perhaps the next decade will see significant progress in this important area.

REFERENCES

Adams CWM: Pathology of multiple sclerosis: progression of the lesion. Br Med Bull 33:15–19, 1977

Anzola GP, Bevilacqua L, Cappa SF, et al: Neuropsychological assessment in patients with relapsing-remitting multiple sclerosis and mild functional impairment: correlation with magnetic resonance imaging. J Neurol Neurosurg Psychiatry 53:142–145, 1990

Baumhefner RW, Tourtellotte WW, Syndulko K, et al: Quantitative multiple sclerosis plaque assessment with magnetic resonance imaging: its correlation with clinical parameters, evoked potentials, and intra-blood-brain barrier IgG synthesis. Arch Neurol 47:19–26, 1990

Beatty PA, Gange JJ: Neuropsychological aspects of multiple sclerosis. J Nerv Ment Dis 164:42–50, 1977

Beatty WW, Goodkin DE: Screening for cognitive impairment in multiple sclerosis: an evaluation of the Mini-Mental State Exam. Arch Neurol 47:297–301, 1990

Beatty WW, Goodkin DE, Monson N, et al: Anterograde and retrograde amnesia in patients with chronic progressive multiple sclerosis. Arch Neurol 45:611–619, 1988

Beatty WW, Goodkin DE, Beatty PA, et al: Frontal lobe dysfunction and memory impairment in patients with chronic progressive multiple sclerosis. Brain Cogn 11:73–86, 1989

Beatty WW, Goodkin DE, Hertsgaard D, et al: Clinical and demographic predictors of cognitive performance in multiple sclerosis: do diagnostic type, disease duration, and disability matter? Arch Neurol 47:305–308, 1990

Ben-Yishay Y, Diller L: Cognitive rehabilitation, in Rehabilitation of the Head Injured Adult. Edited by Rosenthal M, Griffith ER, Bond MR, et al. Philadelphia, PA, FA Davis, 1983, pp 367–380

Bertrando P, Maffei C, Ghezzi A: A study of neuropsychological alterations in multiple sclerosis. Acta Psychiatr Belg 83:13–21, 1983

Brainin M, Goldenberg G, Ahlers C, et al: Structural brain correlates of anterograde memory deficits in multiple sclerosis. J Neurol 235:362–365, 1988

Brooks DJ, Leenders KL, Head G, et al: Studies on regional cerebral oxygen utilisation and cognitive function in multiple sclerosis. J Neurol Neurosurg Psychiatry 47:1182–1191, 1984

Brownell B, Hughes JF: The distribution of plaques in the cerebrum in multiple sclerosis. J Neurol Neurosurg Psychiatry 25:315–320, 1962

Buschke H: Selective reminding for analysis of memory and learning. Journal of Verbal Learning and Verbal Behavior 12:543–550, 1973

Caine ED, Bamford KA, Schiffer RB, et al: A controlled neuropsychological comparison of Huntington's disease and multiple sclerosis. Arch Neurol 43:249–254, 1986

Callanan MM, Logsdail SJ, Ron MA, et al: Cognitive impairment in patients with clinically isolated lesions of the type seen in multiple sclerosis: a psychometric and MRI study. Brain 112:361–374, 1989

Carroll M, Gates R, Roldan F: Memory impairment in multiple sclerosis. Neuropsychologia 22:297–302, 1984

Charcot JM: Lectures on the diseases of the nervous system delivered at La Salpêtrière. London, New Syndenham Society, 1877

Cottrell SS, Wilson SAK: The affective symptomatology of disseminated sclerosis: a study of 100 cases. Journal of Neurology and Psychopathology 7:1–30, 1926

De Smedt L, Severts M, Geutjens J, et al: Intellectual impairment in multiple sclerosis, in Immunological and Clinical Aspects of Multiple Sclerosis. Edited by Gonsette RF, Delmotte P. Lancaster, England, MTP Press, 1984, pp 342–345

Filley CM, Heaton RK, Nelson LM, et al: A comparison of dementia in Alzheimer's disease and multiple sclerosis. Arch Neurol 46:157–161, 1989

Fischer JS: Using the Wechsler Memory Scale-Revised to detect and characterize memory deficits in multiple sclerosis. Clinical Neuropsychologist 2:149–172, 1988

Folstein MF, Folstein SE, McHugh PR: Mini-Mental State: a practical method for grading the cognitive state of patients for the clinician. J Psychiatr Res 12:189–198, 1975

Franklin GM, Heaton RK, Nelson LM, et al: Correlation of neuropsychological and MRI findings in chronic/progressive multiple sclerosis. Neurology 38:1826–1829, 1988

Franklin GM, Nelson LM, Filley CM, et al: Cognitive loss in multiple sclerosis: case reports and review of the literature. Arch Neurol 46:162–167, 1989

Grant I, McDonald WI, Trimble MR, et al: Deficient learning and memory in early and middle phases of multiple sclerosis. J Neurol Neurosurg Psychiatry 47:250–255, 1984

Haughton VM, Ho K-C, Williams AL, et al: CT detection of demyelinated plaques in multiple sclerosis. American Journal of Roentgenology 132:213–215, 1979

Heaton RK, Nelson LM, Thompson DS, et al: Neuropsychological findings in relapsing-remitting and chronic-progressive multiple sclerosis. J Consult Clin Psychol 53:103–110, 1985

Huber SJ, Paulson GW, Shuttleworth EC, et al: Magnetic resonance imaging correlates of dementia in multiple sclerosis. Arch Neurol 44:732–736, 1987

Huckman MS, Fox JH, Topel J: The validity of criteria for the evaluation of cerebral atrophy by computed tomography. Radiology 116:85–92, 1975

Ivnik RJ: Neuropsychological test performance as a function of the duration of MS-related symptomatology. J Clin Psychiatry 39:304–307, 1978

Jacobs L, Kinkel WR, Polachini I, et al: Correlations of nuclear magnetic resonance imaging, computerized tomography, and clinical profiles in multiple sclerosis. Neurology 36:27–34, 1986

Jacobson JT, Deppe U, Murray TJ: Dichotic paradigms in multiple sclerosis. Ear Hearing 4:311–317, 1983

Jambor KL: Cognitive functioning in multiple sclerosis. Br J Psychiatry 115:765–775, 1969

Joffe RT, Lippert GP, Gray TA, et al: Mood disorder and multiple sclerosis. Arch Neurol 44:376–378, 1987

Johnson RT, Katzman R, McGeer E, et al: Report of the panel on inflammatory, demyelinating and degenerative diseases (Report No 79-1916). Washington, DC, US Department of Health, 1979

Katz MM, Lyerly SB: Methods of measuring adjustment and behavior in the community, I: rationale, description, discriminative validity, and scale development. Psychol Rep 13:503–535, 1963

Kurtzke JF: Rating neurologic impairment in multiple sclerosis: an Expanded Disability Status Scale (EDSS). Neurology 33:1444–1452, 1983

Kurtzke JF, Beebe GW, Nagler B, et al: Studies on the natural history of multiple sclerosis, V: long-term survival in young men. Arch Neurol 22:215–225, 1970

Leo GJ, Rao SM: Effects of intravenous physostigmine and lecithin on memory loss in multiple sclerosis: report of a pilot study. Journal of Neurological Rehabilitation 2:123–129, 1988

Litvan I, Grafman J, Vendrell P, et al: Multiple memory deficits in patients with multiple sclerosis: exploring the working memory system. Arch Neurol 45:607–610, 1988a

Litvan I, Grafman J, Vendrell P, et al: Slowed information processing in multiple sclerosis. Arch Neurol 45:281–285, 1988b

Lukes SA, Crooks LE, Aminoff MJ, et al: Nuclear magnetic resonance imaging in multiple sclerosis. Ann Neurol 13:592–601, 1983

Lyon-Caen O, Jouvent R, Hauser S, et al: Cognitive function in recent-onset demyelinating diseases. Arch Neurol 43:1138–1141, 1986

Marsh G: Disability and intellectual function in multiple sclerosis. J Nerv Ment Dis 168:758–762, 1980

Medaer R, Nelissen E, Appel B, et al: Magnetic resonance imaging and cognitive functioning in multiple sclerosis. J Neurol 235:86–89, 1987

Minden SL, Schiffer RB: Affective disorders in multiple sclerosis: review and recommendations for clinical research. Arch Neurol 47:98–104, 1990

Minden SL, Moes EJ, Orav J, et al: Memory impairment in multiple sclerosis. J Clin Exp Neuropsychol 12:566–586, 1990

Nelson LM, Franklin GM, Hamman RF, et al: Referral bias in multiple sclerosis research. J Clin Epidemiol 41:187–192, 1988

Parsons OA, Stewart KD, Arenberg D: Impairment of abstracting ability in multiple sclerosis. J Nerv Ment Dis 125:221–225, 1957

Peyser JM, Edwards KR, Poser CM, et al: Cognitive function in patients with multiple sclerosis. Arch Neurol 37:577–579, 1980

Peyser JM, Rao SM, LaRocca NG, et al: Guidelines for neuropsychological research in multiple sclerosis. Arch Neurol 47:94–97, 1990

Powell HC, Lampert PW: Pathology of multiple sclerosis. Neurol Clin 1:631–644, 1983

Rabins PV, Brooks BR, O'Donnell P, et al: Structural brain correlates of emotional disorder in multiple sclerosis. Brain 109:585–597, 1986

Rao SM: Neuropsychology of multiple sclerosis: a critical review. J Clin Exp Neuropsychol 8:503–542, 1986

Rao SM (ed): Neurobehavioral Aspects of Multiple Sclerosis. New York, Oxford University Press, 1990a

Rao SM: Neuroimaging correlates of cognitive dysfunction, in Neurobehavioral Aspects of Multiple Sclerosis. Edited by Rao SM. New York, Oxford University Press, 1990b, pp 118–135

Rao SM: Multiple sclerosis, in Subcortical Dementia. Edited by Cummings JL. New York, Oxford University Press, 1990c, pp 164–180

Rao SM, Hammeke TA: Hypothesis testing in patients with chronic progressive multiple sclerosis. Brain Cogn 3:94–104, 1984

Rao SM, Leo GJ: Mood disorder in MS (letter). Arch Neurol 45:247–248, 1988

Rao SM, Hammeke TA, McQuillen MP, et al: Memory disturbance in chronic progressive multiple sclerosis. Arch Neurol 41:625–631, 1984

Rao SM, Glatt S, Hammeke TA, et al: Chronic progressive multiple sclerosis: relationship between cerebral ventricular size and neuropsychological impairment. Arch Neurol 42:678–682, 1985

Rao SM, Hammeke TA, Speech TJ: Wisconsin Card Sorting Test performance in relapsing-remitting and chronic-progressive multiple sclerosis. J Consult Clin Psychol 55:263–265, 1987

Rao SM, St. Aubin-Faubert P, Leo GJ: Information processing speed in patients with multiple sclerosis. J Clin Exp Neuropsychol 11:471–477, 1989a

Rao SM, Bernardin L, Leo GJ, et al: Cerebral disconnection in multiple sclerosis: relationship to atrophy of the corpus callosum. Arch Neurol 46:918–920, 1989b

Rao SM, Leo GJ, St. Aubin-Faubert P: On the nature of memory disturbance in multiple sclerosis. J Clin Exp Neuropsychol 11:699–712, 1989c

Rao SM, Leo GJ, Haughton VM, et al: Correlation of magnetic resonance imaging with neuropsychological testing in multiple sclerosis. Neurology 39:161–166, 1989d

Rao SM, Leo GJ, Ellington I, et al: Cognitive dysfunction in multiple sclerosis, II: impact on social functioning. Neurology 41:692–696, 1991a

Rao SM, Leo GJ, Bernardin L, et al: Cognitive dysfunction in multiple sclerosis, I: frequency, patterns, and prediction. Neurology 41:685–691, 1991b

Raven JC: Guide to the Standard Progressive Matrices. London, HK Lewis, 1960

Rey A: L'examine Clinique en Psychologie. Paris, Presses Univesitaries de France, 1964

Rubens AB, Froehling B, Slater G, et al: Left ear suppression on verbal dichotic tests in patients with multiple sclerosis. Ann Neurol 18:459–463, 1985

Schiffer RB, Wineman NM, Weitkamp LR: Association between bipolar affective disorder and multiple sclerosis. Am J Psychiatry 143:94–95, 1986

Smith A: Symbol Digit Modalities Test. Los Angeles, CA, Western Psychological Services, 1973

Staples D, Lincoln NB: Intellectual impairment in multiple sclerosis and its relation to functional abilities. Rheumatology and Rehabilitation 18:153–160, 1979

Stuss DT, Benson DF: Neuropsychological studies of the frontal lobes. Psychol Bull 95:3–28, 1984

Sugar C, Nadell R: Mental symptoms in multiple sclerosis: a study of 28 cases with review of the literature. J Nerv Ment Dis 98:267–280, 1943

Truelle JL, Palisson E, Gall DLe, et al: Troubles intellectuels et thymiques dans la sclerose en plaques. Rev Neurol 143:595–601, 1987

Unverzagt F, Rao SM, Antuono P: Oral physostigmine in the treatment of memory loss in multiple sclerosis (abstract). J Clin Exp Neuropsychol 13:74, 1991

van den Burg W, van Zomeren AH, Minderhoud JM, et al: Cognitive impairment in patients with multiple sclerosis and mild physical disability. Arch Neurol 44:494–501, 1987

Vowels LM, Gates GR: Neuropsychological findings, in Multiple Sclerosis: Psychological and Social Aspects. Edited by Simons AF. London, Heinemann, 1984, pp 82–90

Wechsler D: Wechsler Adult Intelligence Scale. New York, Psychological Corporation, 1955

Wechsler D: Wechsler Memory Scale. New York, Psychological Corporation, 1956

Wechsler D: Wechsler Adult Intelligence Scale—Revised. San Antonio, TX, Psychological Corporation, 1981

Whitlock FA, Siskind MM: Depression as a major symptom of multiple sclerosis. J Neurol Neurosurg Psychiatry 43:861–865, 1980

Willoughby EW, Paty DW: Brain imaging in multiple sclerosis, in Neurobehavioral Aspects of Multiple Sclerosis. Edited by Rao SM. New York, Oxford University Press, 1990, pp 37–62

Young AC, Saunders J, Ponsford JR: Mental change as an early feature of multiple sclerosis. J Neurol Neurosurg Psychiatry 39:1008–1013, 1976

Young IR, Hall AS, Pallis CA, et al: Nuclear magnetic resonance imaging of the brain in multiple sclerosis. Lancet 2:1063–1066, 1981

Zung WK: A self-rating depression scale. Arch Gen Psychiatry 12:63–70, 1965

Chapter 4

Role of Genetic Factors for the Autoimmune Pathogenesis of Multiple Sclerosis

Roland Martin, M.D., Henry F. McFarland, M.D.

Multiple sclerosis (MS) is the most frequent demyelinating disorder in Northern America and Europe. It can involve every part of the central nervous system (CNS). The lesions are characterized by loss of myelin, with generally intact axons (Prineas 1985). The regions of demyelination are often well demarcated, both grossly and microscopically, from areas with intact myelin leading to the appearance of plaques (Prineas 1985). Frequently, particularly in newer lesions, increased cellularity, predominantly macrophages but some T cells, is seen at the leading edge of demyelination. The lesions are most often perivascular and contain lymphocytic infiltrates in new or acute lesions. There is a predilection for MS plaques in the periventricular areas of the brain, but they can also occur throughout the white matter of the CNS. The inflammatory nature of the lesions in MS has suggested an immunopathological mechanism as a cause of the disease (Prineas 1985).

The hallmark of MS is its highly variable clinical course. Most often, the disease starts with acute exacerbations such as loss of vision or sensation followed by recovery, often complete within a period of weeks. In many patients the relapsing-remitting course eventually evolves into a chronic progressive one in which worsening occurs without clear-cut episodes. Some patients, however, will continue to have a relapsing-remitting course often with only minimal disability, whereas others may begin initially with

The authors wish to thank E. Cowan, Neuroimmunology Branch, National Institute of Neurological Disorders and Stroke, National Institutes of Health, for critical discussion of the manuscript.

a progressive, more severe course. It is impossible to predict the future course of the disease in any particular patient.

Presently, there is no laboratory test or imaging study that is specific for MS; the diagnosis continues to be based primarily on clinical criteria. Necessary for diagnosis is evidence of lesions of the CNS separated in both location and time and without an alternative explanation. Recent guidelines allow the use of diagnostic procedures such as visual, auditory, or somatosensory evoked responses and magnetic resonance imaging (MRI) to provide evidence for the second lesion. The diagnosis of MS is also supported by changes in the cerebrospinal fluid (CSF), which include elevated immunoglobulin (IgG) levels, abnormal IgG index, and oligoclonal Ig banding on electrophoresis (Tourtellotte 1985). The MRI has now become the single most useful test in evaluating patients with MS. The lesions of MS appear as hyperintense or bright white matter lesions on T2- or proton-weighted images. Areas of enhancement on T1-weighted images following the administration of gadolinium diethylenetriamine pentaacetic acid (DTPA) represent a breakdown in the blood-brain barrier and are interpreted as new or acute lesions. Importantly, hyperintense lesions on T2-weighted images are not diagnostic for MS. They may occur in other diseases such as CNS vasculitides and can be seen in older individuals, especially those with hypertension or diabetes mellitus. Consequently, caution must be used in interpretation of MRI findings if the clinical findings are not consistent with MS or if they could be explained by alternative diagnoses.

The etiology of MS is still unknown, but both genetic and environmental factors have been postulated to contribute to its pathogenesis. Because of the parallels with experimental animal models for demyelinating diseases such as experimental allergic encephalomyelitis (EAE), it is widely believed that MS is an autoimmune disease mediated by T lymphocytes specific for antigens of the nervous system (Raine 1985). The target antigen within the CNS against which the autoimmune response is directed has not yet been identified. Because susceptibility to EAE is closely linked to the genetic background of the animal, similar genetic influences have been sought in MS (Fritz and McFarlin 1989). Epidemiological studies have suggested an environmental factor in the etiology of MS. Despite many reports of isolations of various infectious agents, particularly viruses, none have withstood rigorous testing (Johnson 1985). Although several experimental models exist in which an EAE-like disease is triggered or induced by infections, these also seem to be under genetic control (Watanabe et al. 1983). Consequently, infections, possibly with common viruses, may contribute to the etiology of the disease.

Evidence for a genetic influence in MS comes from several sources. It has long been recognized that family members of patients with MS seem to have a higher risk of developing the disease than those without a family history of MS (Myrianthopoulos 1985). The risk is even greater in identical twins of individuals with MS. In addition, the disease appears to have greater prevalence in some ethnic groups, whereas in others it is almost nonexistent. Identification of the gene(s) influencing susceptibility has been difficult. Most evidence now suggests that multiple genes may be involved. Because an immunopathological basis for MS has been postulated, attention has focused on genes that influence the immune response, such as those for human leukocyte antigens (HLA) and the T-cell receptor (TCR). In this chapter, we discuss the findings supporting the relationship between these genes, as well as how the products of these genes may contribute to the cause of the disease.

POPULATION STUDIES

Different prevalence rates for MS in various ethnic groups have been reported in several studies (Francis et al. 1987; Hawkins and Kee 1988; Sibley et al. 1989). In North American and northern European populations, which are primarily of Caucasian origin, the prevalence rate ranges between 10 and 130 per 100,000, with a mean of approximately 60 per 100,000 (Kurtzke 1980; Sibley et al. 1989). A considerably higher prevalence rate ranging from 137 to 178 per 100,000 is found in areas such as Northern Ireland or northeast Scotland (Francis et al. 1987; Hawkins and Kee 1988).

In general, the prevalence rates decrease with latitude on both hemispheres; this has been interpreted as an argument favoring environmental influences. Exceptions, however, observed in a number of ethnic groups, show that genetic predisposition, as well as exogenous factors, play a role. A low prevalence rate is, for example, seen not only in Japan (2 per 100,000) (Detels et al. 1983), but also in Japanese people living in Hawaii or on the Pacific coast of the United States. Similarly, the rate found in Hungarians of Caucasian descent is 37 per 100,000, but it is only 2 per 100,000 in Hungarian gypsies (Palffy 1983). A low prevalence rate is also documented for other distinct ethnic groups such as Hutterites, Yakut, Inuit, and Bantu (Waksman and Reynolds 1984). Although these differences are striking, they may be at least partly caused by differing life-styles such as nutrition or by other environmental factors. Further support for environmental factors stems from the description of epidemics of MS on the Faeroe Islands (Kurtzke and Hyllestad 1979).

FAMILY AND TWIN STUDIES

Family studies have been applied to identify genetic components, versus environmental factors, that may influence susceptibility to MS. Sadovnick et al. (1988) reported that about 19% of MS patients from British Columbia had one or more affected family members. Investigations conducted in other areas with a high prevalence of MS had comparable results, with familial rates between 12.9% and 17.5% (Ebers 1983; Gudmundsson 1971; Sadovnick and MacLeod 1981). Most of these studies were based on the clinical diagnosis of MS. If laboratory techniques such as the examination of the CSF and MRI scans and evoked potentials were included in the assessment of affected family members, it is likely that even higher rates would be obtained.

Studies during the last decade have documented that individuals with certain HLA types carry higher risks for specific autoimmune diseases, such as diabetes mellitus and rheumatoid arthritis. Consequently, most family studies have focused on the segregation of HLA haplotypes in affected and unaffected family members (Haile et al. 1981; Tiwari et al. 1980). The data obtained from pooled pedigrees derived from previously published families were used for linkage and sibling pair analysis. Several studies demonstrated a tight linkage between MS and certain HLA alleles in some families, particularly those expressing HLA-B7 and -DR2, confirming the strong association of HLA-B7 and -DR2 that had been documented by population studies (see, Tiwari and Terasaki 1985). Taken together, the studies of linkage of MS with HLA antigens suggested the involvement of one genetic and one environmental determinant or two genetic determinants, one of which was closely linked to HLA-B7 and -DR2 in pedigrees expressing those HLA determinants. No conclusive linkage with HLA could be demonstrated in families lacking HLA-B7 or -DR2 (Ho et al. 1982).

The role of genetic influence was also studied by sibling pair analysis using families with two or more affected members. Because this approach only considers affected siblings, it makes no assumptions about the mode of inheritance and is uninfluenced by the penetrance of the disease phenotype, age at onset, or the existence of subclinical disease. The number of shared phenotypes in a sample of 100 sibling pairs studied by Stewart et al. (1981) was interpreted as supporting linkage of a MS susceptibility gene to HLA. These findings, however, were not unequivocally confirmed by other reports. A study of 40 sibling pairs by Ebers et al. (1982) failed to show numbers of shared haplotypes higher than those expected, even when DR2-expressing pairs were analyzed separately.

Difficulties of interpretation and inconsistencies in results derived from family studies may be due to the fact that pooled data from the literature were frequently used. Because there is no specific diagnostic test for MS and the diagnosis in some families was established on the basis of history alone, other disease entities could be included in the pooled data. Although family studies have failed to demonstrate a clear linkage between disease and HLA, they have suggested that two separate genes may be involved and that one may be closely linked to the HLA gene complex on chromosome 6, particularly in families expressing HLA-DR2. Importantly, the family studies indicate that a single gene encoding susceptibility to MS does not exist and raise the possibility that multiple genes, each with only partial influence on susceptibility, may be involved.

The magnitude of the genetic influence in MS suggested by family studies has been further examined in twins. Even if multiple genes influence susceptibility, their importance should be reflected in the degree of concordance in monozygotic (MZ) twins versus that in dizygotic (DZ) twins. If genetic makeup alone accounted for disease, there should be 100% concordance in MZ twins. If genetic factors represented one component of a multifactorial process, concordance in MZ twins would be less than 100%, depending on the importance of the genetic influence, but still greater than that seen in DZ twins.

Several studies of twins have been undertaken, using differing methodology and with somewhat varying results (Currier and Eldridge 1982; Ebers et al. 1986; Heltberg and Holm 1982; Kinnunen et al. 1988; MacKay and Myrianthopoulos 1966; Williams et al. 1980). Although all studies have indicated higher concordance rates for MZ twins than for DZ twins, the magnitude has differed considerably.

In a study (McFarland et al. 1984) of 30 twin sets referred to the National Institutes of Health after advertisement, both twins in 24 of the sets could be classified as having either definite or probable MS, or not having MS. Of these 24 sets (12 MZ and 12 DZ), 50% of the MZ sets were concordant and 17% of the DZ sets were concordant. This study may have overestimated concordance because of the ascertainment bias; there is an increased chance of ascertaining concordant twins by advertisement (Smith 1974). However, follow-up of these sets plus 6 additional sets over a period of 6 years demonstrated that 4 MZ sets initially classified as discordant subsequently became concordant (McFarland et al. 1984). None of the DZ sets changed in concordance. An additional three unaffected MZ twins were found to have MRI abnormalities consistent with MS, raising the possibility of subclinical disease and an even greater concordance rate in MZ twins.

A true estimate of concordance would be best derived from a population-based twin study. Several such studies have been conducted (e.g., Heltberg and Holm 1982). The most extensive population-based study thus far was conducted by Ebers et al. (1986), who evaluated all twins included in the Canadian MS clinics. Twenty-seven MZ sets were identified in which at least one twin had MS. Seven of these sets were concordant; only 1 of the 47 DZ sets was concordant. These results confirm the substantial increase in concordance found in MZ twins but also show, based on the concordance of less than 100%, that genetic influence is not sufficient for disease. Based on the comparison of concordance in MZ and DZ twins, it is postulated that multiple genes may influence susceptibility. These studies are older, however, and the investigators were not able to assess subclinical disease, as can be done with the techniques now available (e.g., MRI). Because MZ twins are genetically identical, but can be clinically discordant even when MRI, evoked potentials, and CSF analysis are used to determine concordancy, environmental factors or somatic changes must contribute significantly to disease susceptibility.

HLA AND MS

The HLA gene complex is located on chromosome 6 and consists of four major loci coding for heterodimeric membrane proteins, which are divided into HLA class I (HLA-A, -B, and -C) and HLA class II (HLA-DP, -DQ, and -DR) genes (Figure 4–1). HLA class I antigens are made of β2 microglobulin and an HLA-encoded polymorphic α-chain glycoprotein, whereas HLA class II antigens are made of an α-chain and a more polymorphic β-chain.

HLA-A, -B, -C, -DR, and -DQ antigens are typed by serological techniques, usually with serums from multiparous women. International HLA workshops compare the serums available for each specificity and provide reference serums (Bodmer et al. 1990). For each of these loci, a number of different alleles have been identified to date, and the nomenclature is updated at international HLA workshops (Bodmer et al. 1990). Over recent years, addi-

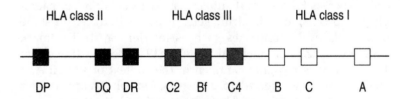

Figure 4–1. Linear map of the human leukocyte antigen (HLA) gene complex region on chromosome 6 (approximately 2 centimorgans). HLA class III (genes encoding complement proteins) are located between HLA class I and class II genes.

tional antiserums have become available, allowing more precise HLA typing and identification of additional antigens. For example, the DR2 serotype can now be split into DRw15 and DRw16. (The *w* stands for *workshop* and indicates that the specificity was derived from reagents described for other DR serotypes.)

Some HLA class II determinants, such as DP, were initially described on the basis of mixed lymphocyte reactions (MLR). Thus, lymphocytes from individuals matched at the serologically defined determinants recognized each other as foreign. Other specificities termed *Dw* were initially identified using MLR. The Dw specificities are not distinct gene products, but rather antigenic portions of either the HLA-DR β-chain or composite reactivities to which HLA-DR, -DP, and -DQ may contribute and that are recognized by T cells. Recently, the amplification of genomic DNA by the polymerase chain reaction (PCR) and analysis of the DNA with sequence-specific oligonucleotides is starting to replace the cellular techniques used for HLA-DP and -Dw typing. Four Dw types associated with DR2 have been described. Strong linkage disequilibrium, meaning that the genes tend to segregate together, exists between the genes encoding the DR and Dw types with those encoding HLA-DQ. The current nomenclature and the associations between some HLA class II antigens are shown in Table 4–1.

The distinction between HLA class I and class II antigens stemmed from the analysis of transplantation reactions, which demonstrated that HLA class I antigen incompatibility was a major factor responsible for graft rejection. This is reflected by the ubiquitous expression of HLA class I antigens on most nucleated cells, whereas HLA class II antigens are detected only on macrophages, B cells, and dendritic cells or can be induced in some other cells by lymphokines such as interferon-γ. In landmark experiments, Zinkernagel and Doherty (1974) demonstrated that T lymphocytes recognize antigen in the context of self-HLA, a mechanism now referred to as *major histocompatibility complex (MHC)* or HLA restriction. HLA class I and class II antigens serve as restriction elements for different lymphocyte populations. It is now well established that T cells recognize antigen that is bound to the HLA class I or class II molecules. Studies (e.g., Bjorkman et al. 1987) of the three-dimensional structure of HLA class I molecules demonstrated that polymorphic parts of the α-chains form a binding groove in which the antigenic peptide is bound. A similar binding groove is thought to be formed by the association of the polymorphic membrane distal domains of HLA class II α- and β-chains. The TCR recognizes both the antigen and portions of the HLA molecule. Cytotoxic T cells that are engaged in the elimination of intracellular pathogens via lysis of infected cells are usually restricted by HLA class I antigens, whereas helper-inducer T cells that secrete lymphokines, such as interleukin-2 or interferon-γ, are restricted by HLA class II antigens. Helper-inducer cells are necessary for providing help for antibody production by B cells and for generation and amplification of class I restricted T cells. In rare instances, class II restricted T cells may also mediate cytotoxic activity.

Over the last two decades, it has become increasingly clear that MHC antigens are crucial in governing T-cell immune responses to foreign antigens, as well as in shaping self-tolerance. Consequently, intensive effort has been directed at examining

Table 4–1. Linkage of HLA-DR types associated with MS in different ethnic groups and HLA-DQ types in linkage disequilibrium with the HLA-DR and -Dw types

HLA-DR type	Split specificities	Dw	DQw
DR2	DRw15	Dw12	DQw6
		Dw2	DQw6
	DRw16	Dw21	DQw5
		Dw22	DQw7
DR4		Dw4	DQw7, DQw8
		Dw10	DQw8
		Dw13A	DQw7, DQw8
		Dw14B	DQw8
		Dw15	DQw4
		Dw"KT2"	
		Dw13B	DQw7, DQw8
		Dw14B	DQw8
DR6	DRw13	Dw18	DQw6
		Dw19	DQw6
		Dw"HAG"	
	DRw14	Dw9	DQw5
		Dw16	DQw7

relationships or associations between HLA and diseases that may be autoimmune in nature, including numerous studies examining HLA makeup in patients with MS.

The first studies reported associations between MS and HLA-A3 and -B7 in North American and northern European Caucasian MS populations (Bertrams and Kuwert 1972, 1976; Jersild et al. 1972; Myrianthopoulos 1985). These results were confirmed in later studies, but further examination including typing for HLA-DR antigens disclosed a stronger association between HLA-DR2 and MS not only in Caucasians but also in black American MS patients (Sibley et al. 1989). As for ethnic groups with lower prevalences of MS, associations with HLA-DR4 were described for Italian (Marrosu et al. 1988) and Arab (Kurdi et al. 1977) MS patients and with HLA-DRw6 for Japanese (Naito et al. 1978) and Mexican (Gorodezky et al. 1986) MS patients.

That other predisposing or even protective factors must exist is pointed out by a report (Palffy 1983) comparing DR2-positive Hungarian MS patients and DR2-positive gypsies living in the same area; the prevalence of MS was much lower in the gypsy population. Some evidence also suggests that HLA makeup may influence clinical course. One study (Hammond et al. 1988) documented an association between a benign relapsing-remitting course of MS and HLA-A3, -B7, and -DR2 and severe chronic progressive disease with HLA-A1, -B8, and -DR3. Rather than an effect on the clinical course, these findings could indicate that different forms of the disease exist.

An association between MS in Caucasians and HLA-DQw1, which is in close linkage disequilibrium with HLA-DR2, has been described (Francis et al. 1987). This association is stronger than that for HLA-DR2Dw2 and MS. A weaker association between HLA-DPw4 and MS was reported in two Scandinavian studies (Moen et al. 1984; Ødum et al. 1988) and was interpreted as a factor independent from HLA-DR2 because HLA-DP antigens are not in linkage disequilibrium with HLA-DR or -DQ.

With the recent advances in molecular biology, the HLA complex has been extensively examined at the molecular level. The amino acid sequences of the individual HLAs and the structure and nucleic acid sequence of the genes encoding these proteins have been determined. The techniques used for these studies have included the generation of characteristic restriction fragment length polymorphisms (RFLPs), DNA sequencing, and amplification of polymorphic regions of certain HLA genes using sequence-specific oligonucleotides and the PCR.

When DNA derived from DR2-positive MS patients was digested with the enzyme EcoR1 and probed with a DQw1 β-chain complementary DNA (cDNA), similar RFLP patterns were obtained from MS patients and control subjects (Cohen et al. 1984). DR2-positive diabetic patients, however, showed a different pattern. When another enzyme, BamH1, was used, a 12-kilobase (kb) fragment was demonstrated that was able to differentiate DR2-positive MS patients from control subjects. From these data it was concluded that a gene within or close to the HLA-DQ β-chain locus is associated with disease and confers a relative risk of 8.8, if an individual was positive for DR2 and the informative BamH1 fragment.

More recent studies have extended these findings. Heard et al. (1989) digested pooled DNA samples from Northern Ireland and northeast Scotland with 14 restriction enzymes and used five HLA-D region probes (DPα, DPβ, DQα, DQβ, and DRβ) and two TCR probes for Southern blot analysis. DNA from the Scottish population was separated into DR2-positive and -negative pools from both control subjects and MS patients. After digestion with the enzyme Msp1 and hybridization with DQα, a 3.25-kb fragment was detected in 31% of the Scottish MS patients compared to 4% of the control subjects. In addition, the fragment was over-represented in DR2-positive MS patients from both geographic areas. The DQα gene detected by the 3.25-kb Msp1 fragment is not yet identified but occurs in allelic form to DQw1, suggesting that two DQ alleles confer susceptibility for disease.

In another study, Vartdal et al. (1989) investigated 61 Norwegian MS patients by typing with sequence-specific oligonucleotides. Fifty-nine of the 61 (97%) were positive for at least one of the HLA-DR specificities (HLA-DR2, -DR4, or -DRw6), specificities that had previously been observed to be associated with MS in different ethnic groups. These specificities were found to be associated with only a few of the many DQβ chains; particular DQβ genes were in linkage disequilibrium with the relevant DR genes. Further analysis of the associated DQβ1 genes and comparison of the amino acid sequences of their polymorphic regions disclosed that they shared most of their membrane distal portions. Because the polymorphic amino acid residues of the HLA class II α- and β-chain form the antigen-binding groove (Brown et al. 1988), it was hypothesized that the conserved amino acid sequences encoded by DR2-, DR4-, and DRw6-associated DQβ1 genes might bind the putative autoantigen that is involved in the immunopathogenesis of MS. This would explain the association between HLA-DR2, -DR4, and -DRw6 and MS.

Different forms of MS may be genetically distinct entities based on association with serologically defined HLAs (Hammond et al. 1988). Olerup et al. (1989) pursued this question by studying the HLA class II gene polymorphism in 100 Scandinavian MS patients. Taq1-digested DNA was probed with DRβ, DQα, and DQβ cDNA probes. In a group of 74 relapsing-remitting MS patients, a positive association with a DQβ1 RFLP pattern found in DRw17 DQw2 haplotypes was observed. Chronic progressive MS in 26 patients was positively associated with a DQβ1 pattern within DR4 DQw8, DR7 DQw9, and DRw8 DQw4 haplotypes, and negatively associated with a DQβ1 pattern corresponding to the serologically defined specificity, DQw7. Both RFLP patterns that were positively associated with chronic progressive or relapsing-remitting MS were allelic to the HLA-DR2 DQw6 haplotype that also demonstrated a positive association.

From the studies of HLA antigens in MS populations conducted so far, it can be concluded that MS is associated with different HLA-DR antigens in different ethnic groups. According to Vartdal et al. (1989), this may mask the association with HLA-DQβ1 genes that encode shared amino acid sequences that are possibly important for the presentation of an autoantigen. The association with HLA-DQw1 in Caucasians is stronger than that with HLA-DR2 Dw2. The studies by Heard et al. (1989) and Olerup et al. (1989), as well as earlier linkage data, suggest that a second HLA antigen may confer additional risk. Based on the data of Heard et al. (1989), this may be a currently unknown DQα gene or, as described by Olerup et al. (1989), another DQβ1 gene allelic to DQβ1 of the HLA-DR2 Dw2 haplotype. Finally, data by the latter authors indicate that chronic progressive and relapsing-remitting MS may be immunogenetically different diseases.

From their investigation of extended HLA haplotypes in patients with MS, Hauser et al. (1990) concluded that HLA-DR2 confers susceptibility and is not simply a marker for at-risk populations. Because it has been demonstrated that alteration of even single amino acids in the putative antigen-binding groove can affect T-cell recognition of antigen, the question arises whether there is a unique HLA class II allele in MS populations that confers susceptibility. This does not appear to be the case. Cowan et al. (1991) analyzed sequences of cDNAs corresponding to the membrane distal domains of HLA class II antigens derived from MS patients and found no differences compared with those found in the general population.

TCR GENES AND MS

The results of linkage, sibling pair analysis, and twin studies suggested that multiple gene loci may be involved in influencing susceptibility for MS. Because it has been long known that T lymphocytes (thymus-derived lymphocytes) are found in the demyelinating foci of MS and that murine EAE can be transferred into naive animals with encephalitogenic T-cell lines, a current hypothesis is that MS is an autoimmune disease mediated by T cells possibly specific for a neural antigen. T cells use a highly polymorphic heterodimeric receptor molecule (TCR) for the recognition of foreign antigen and self-antigen. Unlike immunoglobulin, TCR genes undergo little somatic mutation, and the analysis of the germline repertoire of patients and control subjects might therefore help to disclose TCR α- and β-chain genes that are involved in the disease process. The reports briefly summarized below focus, however, on the germline TCR repertoire rather than on the TCRs expressed by antigen-specific or infiltrating T cells.

Using Southern blot analysis, Beall et al. (1989) digested DNA derived from 40 patients with definite chronic progressive MS and DNA from 100 control subjects and probed it with cDNAs for the constant region of the β-chain and cDNAs representing members of the described human Vβ gene subfamilies, Vβ1 through Vβ14. Allelic forms of Vβ8, Vβ11, and Cβ defined by RFLP allowed analysis of haplotypes comprising these genes in a group of chronic progressive MS patients and control subjects. One haplotype, designated 23/20/9 on the basis of the respective fragment sizes for Vβ8, Vβ11, and Cβ, was overrepresented in the MS patients; the Vβ8/Vβ11 haplotype 2/25 showed a frequency lower than expected. A relative risk of 3.22 could be assigned for the presence of the haplotype 23/20/9 in DR2-positive Caucasian MS patients compared with DR2-positive Caucasian control subjects, indicating that this TCR haplotype conferred additional risk to develop disease for DR2-positive individuals.

A similar approach was used by Oksenberg et al. (1989) for the study of TCR α-chain alleles associated with MS and myasthenia gravis in Californian and Australian MS patients. DNA from 28 Californian and 48 Australian MS patients was digested with PssI. Using cDNA probes for TCR Vα12.1 and Cα, polymorphic bands sized 6.3 kb and 2.0 kb were obtained with the 6.3-kb probe hybridizing to the variable region and the 2.0-kb probe to the constant region. Based on population and family data, these polymorphic markers are found with frequencies of 0.3 and 0.44 in Californian control subjects. When the frequencies found in MS patients were compared with those obtained from control subjects, the distribution of the 6.3-kb RFLP documented a strong association with disease in Californian but not Australian MS patients (relative risks 10.95 and 2.0, respectively), whereas the 2.0-kb probe was strongly associated with disease in both Californian and Australian MS patients (relative risks 16.53 and 16.4, respectively). These differences were interpreted to reflect geographic and ethnic variations.

In a third study, Seboun et al. (1989) investigated the pattern of inheritance of TCR β-chain genes in the families of 40 sibling pairs concordant for relapsing-remitting MS. Haplotypes were assigned using polymorphic TCR β-chain RFLP in MS sibling pairs. The segregation of these haplotypes was then followed, and the mean number of TCR β-chain haplotypes identical by descent was determined. The mean proportion inherited by MS sibling pairs was significantly higher than expected, whereas the distribution was random when compared with their unaffected siblings. In addition, one RFLP marker detected in HindIII-digested DNA and corresponding to a TCR β-chain gene segment was overrepresented on chromosomes of MS patients compared with those chromosomes inherited by healthy offspring.

The data of all three studies suggest that a gene (or genes) within the TCR complex or a locus in close proximity contribute to the susceptibility to MS. It is likely that with increasing data and improving techniques a more precise association between TCR genes and MS will emerge.

POSSIBLE ROLE OF HLA AND TCR GENES FOR THE AUTOIMMUNE PATHOGENESIS OF MS

From the current understanding of the immune system, it is expected that T lymphocytes are able to recognize virtually any antigen including self-antigens. Several mechanisms have been proposed to generate tolerance against self-structures and thus prevent autoimmune disease. These include the deletion of auto-reactive T-cell clones in the thymus, sequestration of autoantigens such as myelin basic protein (MBP) from the immune response via the blood-brain barrier, and control of self-reactive T cells by suppressive mechanisms acting in the periphery. If MS resembles EAE, in which certain MHC class II genes predispose for disease and the disease is mediated by T cells recognizing a well-defined myelin component, it would be expected that tolerance in healthy individuals would result from both sequestration of the antigen and suppression of myelin-specific T cells. Surprisingly, the existence of T cells specific for brain autoantigens such as MBP can be demonstrated in the mature T-cell repertoire of rodents and humans (Chou et al. 1989; Martin et al. 1990; Pette et al. 1990, Schlüsener and Wekerle 1985). In the rat model system, Schlüsener and Wekerle (1985) also demonstrated that these MBP-specific T cells are potentially encephalitogenic when they are expanded in vitro.

Are such autoimmune T cells important for the pathogenesis of MS, and how does the association of MS with certain HLA and TCR genes relate to this process? In recent years, major advances in the analysis of T-cell recognition of foreign antigen and self-antigen helped to address these questions. It is now clear that T cells respond to antigen only if it is presented in the context of self-MHC structures. In addition, T lymphocytes do not recognize conformational determinants of native proteins, but short oligopeptides that are generated from the mature protein by proteolytic degradation in the antigen-presenting cells. The antigenic peptide is then bound to the antigen-binding groove of MHC class I or class II molecules.

The importance of each of the ligands in the trimolecular complex between TCR, MHC molecule, and antigen has been most extensively studied in EAE (Zamvil and Steinman 1990). It was demonstrated that EAE can only be induced with whole myelin or MBP in mouse and rat strains with appropriate immunogenetic backgrounds. The relevant genes are those for class II molecules identified as MHC-Ia molecules (Fritz and McFarlin 1989). Subsequently, it was shown that short peptides of the MBP molecule contained the encephalitogenic parts but that the region that was encephalitogenic in various species and even strains of animals varied depending on the Ia molecules expressed (Fritz and McFarlin 1989). Interestingly, the analysis of the TCRs expressed by encephalitogenic T cells in various susceptible animal strains disclosed that only a very limited number of variable regions were used, $V\beta8.2$ and $V\alpha4$ in the PL mice, $V\beta8.2$ and $V\alpha2.3$ and $V\alpha4.2$ in B10.PL mice, and $V\beta8.2$ and $V\alpha2$ in Lewis rats (Zamvil and Steinman 1990).

The characterization of the three components of the trimolecular complex involved in the autoimmune process has been used to devise various treatment strategies in EAE. The approaches included 1) tolerization with the autoantigen or autoantigen coupled to carrier cells (Clayton et al. 1989; Kennedy et al. 1990); 2) blockade of MHC class II molecules by modified antigenic peptides that strongly bind to the MHC molecule, but are not recognized by encephalitogenic T cells (Wraith et al. 1989); 3) vaccination with whole encephalitogenic T cells or peptides homologous to the TCRs used by these cells (Howell et al. 1989; Vandenbark et al. 1989); and 4) injection of monoclonal antibodies specific for the TCRs expressed by encephalitogenic T cells (Zaller et al. 1990).

If MS is an autoimmune disease, the components of the trimolecular complex responsible for disease have not been identified. Because the relevant antigen or antigens involved in MS are not known, the approaches to the question have been indirect. Although several potential antigens are associated with myelin, attention has focused primarily on MBP and proteolipid protein because both have been shown to induce EAE in experimental animals and both can be isolated from myelin with relative ease. To identify potentially relevant reactivity to either protein, investigators have attempted to identify a component of the immune response to the protein that is unique for patients with MS as compared with control subjects. This approach has had only limited success.

MBP-specific T cells can be easily isolated from the peripheral blood of both MS patients and control subjects, although the frequency may be somewhat greater in MS patients (Chou et al. 1989; Martin et al. 1990; Pette et al. 1990). Current approaches involve examining the response to specific regions or epitopes of the proteins and then identifying the HLA restriction and TCR usage involved in the response to the individual epitope in order to identify a response unique or overrepresented in MS patients. A more detailed analysis of the response to MBP showed that at least two regions of the molecule, one in the middle and one at the C-terminus, are recognized by a large proportion of T cells (Martin et al. 1990).

Ota et al. (1990) described an increase in T cells specific for MBP peptide 84-102 in the blood of MS patients and reported that these cells are restricted by HLA-DR2. Our laboratory (Martin et al. 1992) has mapped the fine specificity of the response to a similar peptide, 87-106, and demonstrated that amino acids 87-96 and 89-99, respectively, represent the core sequences. Finally, it was shown that peptide 87-106 is recognized not only in the context of DR2, but also with DR4 and DRw6.

It should be noted that 97% of Norwegian MS patients have been shown to express HLA-DR2, -DR4, and -DR6 (Vartdal et al. 1989) and that these same HLA-DR molecules had been linked with disease in MS populations of different ethnic backgrounds (as described above). Vartdal et al. (1989) argued that amino acid sequences shared by DQβ1 chains associated with DR2, -DR4, and -DR6 might be involved in the presentation of a target autoantigen of MS. However, our results indicate that the response to MBP peptide 87-106 is entirely DR restricted. Other investigators (e.g., Chou et al. 1989; Ota et al. 1990) have identified only occasional MBP reactive T cells that are HLA-DQ restricted; almost all have been found to be HLA-DR restricted (Martin et al. 1990; Pette et al. 1990). It remains possible that a relevant HLA-DQ–restricted MBP response has been overlooked or that the relevant antigen is not MBP. Considerable attention has also been focused on the TCRs employed by MBP-specific T cells. A shared Vβ or VDJ sequence similar to that found in some rodents would strengthen the association between MBP reactive T cells and MS. Wucherpfennig et al. (1990) found an overrepresentation of Vβ17 expression in T-cell lines specific for MBP peptide 84-102.

More recently, Ben-Nun et al. (1991) described a limited TCR heterogeneity within individuals, but no evidence of restricted usage between individuals. This result would not be unexpected even if restricted TCR usage was associated with MS because humans are so highly diverse. However, another recent report (Kotzin et al. 1991) described an overusage of Vβ5.1 and Vβ6.2 in MBP reactive T-cell lines. The explanation for these differences is not known, but together the results of the various studies suggest a significant degree of heterogeneity in TCR Vβ usage in MS.

Considerable progress has been made in the understanding of the pathogenesis of experimental autoimmune diseases. The predisposing genetic factors that are primarily located in the MHC class II gene complex have been characterized and shown to be the ligands involved in the recognition of relevant target autoantigens. Although MS also shows an association with certain HLA class II genes, it is still uncertain to what extent they contribute to the pathogenesis. Because of the genetic diversity of humans, it is possible that various HLA molecules and TCR genes may allow an encephalitogenic response to a particular neural antigen or that various portions of MBP or other myelin proteins may be encephalitogenic in different individuals depending on their HLA and TCR makeup. If either of these hypotheses is true, identification of the relevant components of the trimolecular complex in human demyelinating disease may be difficult.

In addition to genes for HLA and TCR, it is possible that other genes could also affect susceptibility. Associations with an allotype, GM, occurring in the heavy chain of immunoglobulin (Pandey et al. 1981) and with the genotype for alpha-1 antitrypsin (McCombe et al. 1985) have been described but remain controversial. Boylan et al. (1990) found a DNA length polymorphism 5' to the MBP gene associated with MS. Other relevant genes could involve the ones regulating lymphokine production. Multiple lymphokines, such as interleukin-1, interleukin-2, interleukin-6, transforming growth factor beta (TGF-β), tumor necrosis factor (TNF), and interferon-γ, can have profound effects on the immune response, either by acting directly on T cells or B cells or by effecting the expression of HLA class II molecules necessary for induction of the immune response. In addition, lymphokines such as TNF have been found to be capable of producing demyelination. The gene coding for TNF is located within the HLA complex on chromosome 6. Little is known about genetic diversity involved in the regulation of these substances. Many other genes could also contribute to susceptibility to a disease such as MS.

The past several years have seen tremendous advances in the technologies available for studying genetic influences in human diseases. The availability of these newer and more powerful techniques together with appropriate clinical material, such as well-defined multiplex families, provide considerable hope that the genetic link in MS will give the needed clue to the cause of the disease.

REFERENCES

Beall SS, Concannon P, Charmley P, et al: The germline repertoire of T cell receptor β-chain genes in patients with chronic progressive multiple sclerosis. J Neuroimmunol 21:59–66, 1989

Ben-Nun A, Libiau RS, Cohen L, et al: Restricted receptor Vβ gene usage by myelin basic protein-specific T cell clones in multiple sclerosis: predominant genes vary in individuals. Proc Natl Acad Sci U S A 88:2466–2469, 1991

Bertrams J, Kuwert E: HLA antigen frequencies in multiple sclerosis. European Journal of Neurology 7:74–79, 1972

Bertrams J, Kuwert E: Association of histocompatibility haplotype HLA-A3-B7 with multiple sclerosis. J Immunol 117:1906–1912, 1976

Bjorkman P, Saper M, Samraoui B, et al: The foreign antigen binding site and T cell recognition regions of class I histocompatibility antigens. Nature 329:512–518, 1987

Bodmer JG, Marsh SGE, Parham P, et al: Nomenclature for factors of the HLA system, 1989. Hum Immunol 28:326–342, 1990

Boylan KB, Takahashi N, Paty DW, et al: DNA length polymorphism 5′ to the myelin basic protein gene is associated with multiple sclerosis. Ann Neurol 27:291–297, 1990

Brown JH, Jardetzky T, Saper MA, et al: A hypothetical model of the foreign antigen binding site of class II histocompatibility molecules. Nature 332:845–849, 1988

Chou YK, Vainiene M, Whitham R, et al: Response of human T lymphocyte lines to myelin basic protein: association of dominant epitopes with HLA class II restriction molecules. J Neurosci Res 23:207–216, 1989

Clayton JP, Gammon GM, Ando DG, et al: Peptide-specific prevention of experimental allergic encephalomyelitis. J Exp Med 69:1681–1691, 1989

Cohen D, Cohen O, Marcadet A, et al: Class II HLA-DC b-chain DNA restriction fragments differentiate among HLA-DR2 individuals in insulin-dependent diabetes and multiple sclerosis. Proc Natl Acad Sci U S A 81:1774–1778, 1984

Cowan EP, Pierce ML, McFarland HF, et al: HLA-DR and -DQ allelic sequences in multiple sclerosis patients are identical to those found in the general population. Hum Immunol 32:203–210, 1991

Currier RD, Eldridge R: Possible risk factors in multiple sclerosis as found in a national twin study. Arch Neurol 39:140–144, 1982

Detels R, Visscher B, Malmgren R, et al: Frequency and patterns of multiple sclerosis among Japanese-Americans, in Multiple Sclerosis East and West. Edited by Kuroiwa Y, Kurland LT. Basel, Switzerland, Karger, 1983, pp 171–177

Ebers GC: Genetic factors in multiple sclerosis. Neurol Clin 1:645–654, 1983

Ebers GC, Paty DW, Stiller CR, et al: HLA-typing in multiple sclerosis sibling pairs. Lancet 1:88–90, 1982

Ebers GC, Buhman DE, Sadovnick AD, et al: A population-based study of multiple sclerosis in twins. N Engl J Med 315:1638–1642, 1986

Francis DA, Batchelor JR, McDonald WI, et al: Multiple sclerosis in Northeast Scotland. An association with HLA-DQw1. Brain 110:181–196, 1987

Fritz R, McFarlin DE: Encephalitogenic epitopes of myelin basic protein (volume edited by Sercarz E). Chem Immunol 46:101–125, 1989

Gorodezky C, Najera R, Rangel BE, et al: Immunogenetic profile of multiple sclerosis in Mexicans. Hum Immunol 16:364–374, 1986

Gudmundsson KR: Clinical studies of multiple sclerosis in Iceland. Acta Neurol Scand Suppl 48:1–78, 1971

Haile RW, Iselius L, Hodge SE, et al: Segregation and linkage analysis of 40 multiplex multiple sclerosis families. Hum Hered 31:252–258, 1981

Hammond SR, English D, Dewtit C, et al: The clinical profile of MS in Australia: a comparison between medium-frequency and high-frequency prevalence zones. Neurology 38:980–986, 1988

Hauser SL, Fleischnick E, Weiner HL, et al: Extended major histocompatibility complex haplotypes in patients with multiple sclerosis. Neurology 39:275–277, 1990

Hawkins SA, Kee F: Updated epidemiological studies of multiple sclerosis in Northern Ireland (abstract). J Neurol 235 (suppl):86, 1988

Heard RNS, Cullen C, Middleton D, et al: An allelic cluster of DQa restriction fragments is associated with multiple sclerosis: evidence that a second haplotype may influence disease susceptibility. Hum Immunol 25:111–123, 1989

Heltberg A, Holm NV: Concordance in twins and recurrence in sibships in multiple sclerosis (letter). Lancet 1:1068, 1982

Ho H, Tiwari JC, Haile W, et al: HLA-linked and unlinked determinants of multiple sclerosis. Immunogenetics 15:13–29, 1982

Howell MD, Winters ST, Olee T, et al: Vaccination against experimental allergic encephalomyelitis with T cell receptor peptides. Science 246:668–670, 1989

Jersild C, Svejgard A, Fog T: HLA antigens and multiple sclerosis. Lancet 1:1240–1241, 1972

Johnson RT: Viral aspects of multiple sclerosis, in Handbook of Clinical Neurology, Vol 47. Edited by Vinken PJ, Bruyn GW, Klawans HC; coedited by Koestner JC. New York, Elsevier Science, 1985, pp 319–336

Kennedy MK, Tan L-J, Dal Canto MC, et al: Regulation of the effector stages of experimental autoimmune encephalomyelitis via neuro-antigen-specific tolerance induction. J Immunol 145:117–126, 1990

Kinnunen E, Juntunen J, Ketonen L, et al: Genetic susceptibility to multiple sclerosis: a co-twin study of a nationwide series. Arch Neurol 45:1108–1111, 1988

Kotzin BL, Satyanarayana K, Yuan KC, et al: Preferential T-cell receptor β-chain gene usage in myelin basic protein-reactive T-cell clones from patients with multiple sclerosis. Proc Natl Acad Sci U S A 88:9161-9165, 1991

Kurdi A, Ayesh I, Abdallat A, et al: Different B-lymphozyte alloantigens associated with multiple sclerosis in Arabs and Northern Europeans. Lancet 1:1123–1125, 1977

Kurtzke JF: Epidemiologic contributions to multiple sclerosis: an overview. Neurology 30:61–79, 1980

Kurtzke JF, Hyllestad K: Multiple sclerosis in the Faroe Islands, I: clinical and epidemiological features. Ann Neurol 5:6–21, 1979

MacKay RP, Myrianthopoulos NC: Multiple sclerosis in twins and their relatives. Arch Neurol 15:449–462, 1966

Marrosu HG, Muntoni F, Murru MR, et al: Sardinian multiple sclerosis is associated with HLA-DR4: a serological and molecular analysis. Neurology 38:1749–1753, 1988

Martin R, Jaraquemada D, Flerlage M, et al: Fine specificity and HLA restriction of myelin basic protein-specific cytotoxic T cells from multiple sclerosis patients and healthy individuals. J Immunol 145:540–548, 1990

Martin R, Utz U, Coligan JE, et al: Diversity in fine specificity and T cell receptor usage of the human CD4+ cytotoxic T cell response specific for the immunodominant myelin basic protein peptide 87-106. J Immunol 148:1359–1366, 1992

McCombe PA, Clark P, Frith JA, et al: Alpha-1 antitrypsin phenotypes in demyelinating diseases: an association between demyelinating disease and the allele Pi M3. Ann Neurol 18:514–516, 1985

McFarland HF, Greenstein J, McFarlin DE, et al: Family and twin studies in multiple sclerosis. Ann N Y Acad Sci 436:118–124, 1984

Moen T, Stein R, Bratlie A, et al: Distribution of HLA-SB antigens in multiple sclerosis. Tissue Antigens 24:126–127, 1984

Myrianthopoulos NC: Genetic aspects of multiple sclerosis, in Handbook of Clinical Neurology, Vol 47. Edited by Vinken PJ, Bruyn GW, Klawans HC; coedited by Koestner JC. New York, Elsevier Science, 1985, pp 289–317

Naito S, Kuroiwa Y, Itoyama T, et al: HLA and Japanese MS. Tissue Antigens 12:19–24, 1978

Ødum N, Hyldig-Nielsen JJ, Morling N, et al: HLA-DP antigens are involved in the susceptibility to multiple sclerosis. Tissue Antigens 31:235-237, 1988

Oksenberg JR, Sherritt M, Begovich AB, et al: T-cell receptor $V\alpha$ and $C\alpha$ alleles associated with multiple sclerosis and myasthenia gravis. Proc Natl Acad Sci U S A 86:988–992, 1989

Olerup O, Hillert J, Fredrikson S, et al: Primarily chronic progressive and relapsing/remitting multiple sclerosis: two immunogenetically distinct disease entities. Proc Natl Acad Sci U S A 86:7113–7117, 1989

Ota K, Matsui M, Milford EL, et al: T-cell recognition of an immunodominant myelin basic protein epitope in multiple sclerosis. Nature 346:183–187, 1990

Palffy G: MS in Hungary, including Gypsy population, in Multiple Sclerosis East and West. Edited by Kuroiwa Y, Kurland LT. Basel, Switzerland, Karger, 1983, pp 149–157

Pandey JP, Goust JM, Salier JP, et al: Immunoglobulin G heavy chain (Gm) allotypes in multiple sclerosis. J Clin Invest 67:1797–1800, 1981

Pette M, Fujita K, Kitze B, et al: Myelin basic protein-specific T lymphocyte lines from MS patients and healthy individuals. Neurology 40:1770–1776, 1990

Prineas JW: The neuropathology of multiple sclerosis, in Handbook of Clinical Neurology, Vol 47. Edited by Vinken PJ, Bruyn GW, Klawans HC; coedited by Koestner JC. New York, Elsevier Science, 1985, pp 213–257

Raine CS: Experimental allergic encephalomyelitis and experimental allergic neuritis, in Handbook of Clinical Neurology, Vol 47. Edited by Vinken PJ, Bruyn GW, Klawans HC; coedited by Koestner JC. New York, Elsevier Science, 1985, pp 429–466

Sadovnick AD, MacLeod PMJ: The familial nature of multiple sclerosis: empiric recurrence risks for first-, second- and third-degree relatives of patients. Neurology 31:1039–1041, 1981

Sadovnick AD, Baird PA, Ward RH: Multiple sclerosis: updated risks for relatives. Am J Med Genet 29:533–541, 1988

Schlüsener H, Wekerle H: Autoaggressive T lymphocyte lines recognize the encephalitogenic region of myelin basic protein: in vitro selection from unprimed rat T lymphocyte populations. J Immunol 135:3128–3133, 1985

Seboun E, Robinson MA, Doolittle TH, et al: A susceptibility locus for multiple sclerosis is linked to the T cell receptor β chain complex. Cell 57:1095–1100, 1989

Sibley WA, Poser CM, Alter M: Multiple sclerosis, in Merritt's Textbook of Neurology, 8th Edition. Edited by Rowland LP. Philadelphia, PA, Lea & Febiger, 1989, pp 741–765

Smith C: Concordance in twins: methods and interpretation. Am J Hum Genet 26:454–466, 1974

Stewart GJ, McLeod JG, Basten A, et al: HLA family studies and multiple sclerosis: a common gene, dominantly expressed. Hum Immunol 3:13–29, 1981

Tiwari JL, Terasaki PI: HLA and Disease Associations. New York, Springer-Verlag, 1985, pp 152–167

Tiwari JC, Hodge SE, Terasaki PI, et al: HLA and the inheritance of multiple sclerosis: linkage analysis in 72 pedigrees. Am J Hum Genet 32:103–111, 1980

Tourtellotte WW: The cerebrospinal fluid in multiple sclerosis, in Handbook of Clinical Neurology, Vol 47. Edited by Vinken PJ, Bruyn GW, Klawans HC; coedited by Koestner JC. New York, Elsevier Science, 1985, pp 79–130

Vandenbark AA, Hashim G, Offner H: Immunization with a synthetic T-cell receptor V-region against experimental autoimmune encephalomyelitis. Nature 341:541–544, 1989

Vartdal F, Sollid LM, Vandvik B, et al: Patients with multiple sclerosis carry DQB1 genes which encode shared polymorphic amino acid sequences. Hum Immunol 25:103–110, 1989

Waksman BH, Reynolds WE: Minireview: multiple sclerosis as a disease of immune regulation. Proc Soc Exp Biol Med 175:282–294, 1984

Watanabe R, Wege H, ter Meulen V: Adoptive transfer of EAE-like lesions from rats with coronavirus-induced demyelinating encephalomyelitis. Nature 305:150–152, 1983

Williams A, Elridge R, McFarland HF, et al: Multiple sclerosis in twins. Neurology 30:1139–1147, 1980

Wraith DC, McDevitt HO, Steinman L, et al: T cell recognition as the target for immune intervention in autoimmune disease. Cell 57:709–715, 1989

Wucherpfennig KW, Ota K, Endo N, et al: Shared human T cell receptor Vb usage to immunodominant regions of myelin basic protein. Science 248:1016–1019, 1990

Zaller DM, Osman G, Kanagawa O, et al: Prevention and treatment of murine experimental allergic encephalomyelitis with T cell receptor Vβ-specific antibodies. J Exp Med 171:1943–1955, 1990

Zamvil SS, Steinman L: The T lymphocyte in experimental allergic encephalomyelitis. Ann Rev Immunol 8:579–621, 1990

Zinkernagel RM, Doherty PC: Immunological surveillance against altered self components by sensitized T lymphocytes in lymphocytic choriomeningitis. Nature 251:547–548, 1974

Chapter 5

Current Treatment Strategies and Perspectives of Multiple Sclerosis

Lawrence Jacobs, M.D.,
Frederick E. Munschauer, M.D., and
Patrick Pullicino, M.D.

Multiple Sclerosis (MS) is an autoimmune inflammatory disease confined to the central nervous system (CNS). It is currently believed that MS is caused by an environmental factor (viral) acting on an individual with genetically determined dysimmunity (Rodriguez 1989). Whatever the triggering agent, there is a large body of evidence indicating that MS patients have an abnormal immune response resulting in inflammatory CNS lesions characterized by predominantly perivascular lesions of inflammation, demyelination (axon sparing), and gliosis. The lesions of MS (plaques) can be identified with great sensitivity with magnetic resonance imaging (MRI) (positive in 87%–95% of cases) and with lesser degrees of sensitivity by computed tomography (CT) imaging (positive in approximately 35% of cases) (Figure 5–1).

Epidemiological data (Kurtzke 1980, 1983) support a viral or other environmental factor as the cause of MS. The highest concentration of the disease occurs between 37° and 52° north latitude of the globe. Areas of high prevalence are bordered by areas of medium prevalence, which in turn are surrounded by areas of low prevalence. Migration studies show that individuals moving from one geographic region to another after the first 10–12 years of life will retain the risk for MS of their birthplace in their new environment (Kurtzke 1980, 1983; Kurtzke et al. 1979). This suggests that exposure to the MS agent occurs at a young age and that years or even decades pass before development of symptomatic disease.

To date no virus that is specific or exclusive to MS has been identified. Viral studies in MS using antibody probes and isolation techniques have identified several viruses in MS patients that might conceivably be responsible; the most commonly reported has been measles virus (Haase et al. 1981; terMeulen and Stephenson 1983). The causal relationship of these viruses in MS has never been established with certainty; indeed, the incidence of viral antibodies in MS patients' serum and cerebrospinal fluid (CSF) may not be statistically different from that for non-MS individuals.

The most compelling direct recent evidence supporting a viral etiology of MS comes from our understanding of tropical spastic paraparesis, which presents clinicopathologically in a fashion similar to chronic progressive MS and has been shown to be caused by the retrovirus human T-cell lymphotropic virus type I (HTLV-I) (Gessain et al. 1985). This finding has stimulated a

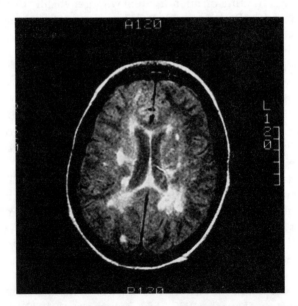

Figure 5–1. Cerebral magnetic resonance image (MRI) scan of patient with multiple sclerosis. Lesions appear as areas of high signal intensities (bright) of cerebral parenchyma predominantly, but not exclusively, in the periventricular regions. T2-weighted image TR2200, TE30.

number of studies on the possible role of retroviruses in MS. Early reports that indicated an association of MS and a retrovirus distinct from, but related to, the known HTLVs were not subsequently substantiated in larger studies (Booss and Kim 1990). Molecular genetic techniques, most remarkably the polymerase chain reaction, are capable of detecting viral genomes in cells of systemic circulation or CSF. This technique has been used in MS patients to probe for a number of DNA and RNA viruses, but none has been reliably or reproducibly identified (Booss and Kim 1990).

Thus the strongest support for viral etiology comes from the epidemiological data, with only subsidiary evidence from viral isolation-antibody studies. It may be impossible to recover the virus responsible for MS. Indeed, as suggested by epidemiological data, an initial viral infection may occur at a young age (Kurtzke 1980, 1983; Kurtzke et al. 1979) and persist long enough for a clone of T or B cells against a CNS antigen to be established, after which all viral material may be cleared by the immune system. Reactivation of these committed immune-cell lines may then mediate CNS inflammatory lesions decades after an initial infection (Khoury et al. 1990).

IMMUNE STATE IN MS

Abnormalities in both humoral and cellular immunity have been identified in MS. High titers of antibodies in the CSF, impaired suppressor-cell function, and impaired effector-cell (natural killer cell) function have all been identified (Kastrukoff et al. 1986; Rice et al. 1983). However, none of these abnormalities is pathognomonic for MS, and as yet the mechanism of the dysimmunity of MS remains unknown.

Disorders of Humoral Immune Response in MS

Disordered B-cell function has been a clinical hallmark of MS since Kabat et al. (1942) first reported elevation of immunoglobulin (IgG) within the CNS of MS patients. The IgG abnormality, combined with oligoclonal bands in the CSF, is a pattern that is characteristic of MS, but not necessarily diagnostic of the disease. Rudick et al. (1986) found intrathecal production of free κ and λ light chain monomers and dimers in the CSF of 10 MS patients but none in the CSF of 14 control subjects; this abnormality is currently believed to be more sensitive and specific for MS than elevated CSF IgG or oligoclonal bands. The presence of CSF free light chains is direct evidence of B-cell dysfunction, either in the regulation of IgG synthesis or in pseudoneoplastic dysfunction (e.g., monoclonal gammopathy). Alternatively, aberrant IgG synthesis could be caused by suppressor T-cell dysfunction as B-cell proliferation and differentiation is regulated by T cells.

Disorders of Cellular Immunity in MS

The most important T-cell dysfunction identified is impaired suppressor-cell function (Paty et al. 1983). The suppressor-cell abnormalities include impaired function of suppressor cells, selective loss of suppressor-inducer cells (CD3+,CD4+, CD45R+), impaired activation of suppressor cells or suppressor-cell subsets, and impaired suppressor-cell maturation (Morimoto et al. 1982). Additionally, circulating natural killer cells have been reported to decrease with exacerbations and also with the occurrence of new lesions on MRI (Oger et al. 1988).

THERAPY

The therapeutic approaches to MS are directed at its inflammation and dysimmunity. Corticosteroids have immunomodulatory as well as anti-inflammatory properties. Oral prednisone, adrenocorticotropic hormone (ACTH), and high-dose intravenous methylprednisolone are all used commonly in the management of MS exacerbations or in active chronic progressive disease.

Conventional Treatment: Exacerbating Disease

Although some agents are effective for exacerbations, no treatment has been shown to modify the overall course of exacerbating MS. The management of exacerbating disease is confounded by the unpredictable nature of exacerbations, which may be separated by months or decades, thus precluding the use of medication on a continuous basis. Therapy for exacerbating disease is currently limited to treatment of acute exacerbations with the objective of reducing the severity and duration of attacks.

ACTH. In the first randomized, placebo-controlled study (Miller et al. 1961), intramuscular ACTH was shown to be significantly better than placebo ($P < .05$) in decreasing exacerbation duration and severity. These results were confirmed nearly a decade later in a larger multicenter study that included 197 patients with relapsing MS (Rose et al. 1970). Patients treated within 8 weeks of an acute relapse with a 2-week course of intramuscular ACTH showed significantly more improvement ($P < .05$) during treatment than did placebo-treated control subjects. Unfortunately, ACTH treatment only reduced the severity and shortened the duration of exacerbations; it did not change the long-term course of the disease. The findings of these seminal studies (Miller et al. 1961; Rose et al. 1970) have withstood the tests of time. After the 1970 study a 10- to 14-day course of intramuscular ACTH became accepted as the standard best treatment for acute exacerbations of MS (Troiano et al. 1990). Predictable, but infrequent, side effects of ACTH treatment include hypertension and peripheral edema caused by its mineralocorticoid activity, mood changes, and insomnia. Only rarely are these side effects severe enough to stop therapy.

Oral prednisone. Like ACTH, oral prednisone has immunomodulatory and anti-inflammatory properties. Advantages over ACTH include less mineralocorticoid effect and the convenience of taking it orally rather than through intramuscular or intravenous injections. Disadvantages include a higher incidence of gastrointestinal side effects. Moreover, several investigators have reported that prednisone is not as effective as ACTH in shortening the duration or severity of exacerbations (Myers 1992).

Prednisone is usually administered in dosages of 40–120 mg/day for 2–3 weeks. Antacids; histamine, subtype 2 (H_2), blockers; or gastric mucosal barriers, such as sucralfate (Carafate), should also be given. Chronic administration is associated with the usual side effects of corticosteroids. Additionally, it has been our experience that neurological deterioration may occur when patients are weaned from chronic steroids despite apparently inactive disease. Therefore, under usual circumstances oral prednisone should not be used in favor of ACTH for treating acute exacerbations.

Intravenous methylprednisolone. Several controlled studies (Abbruzzese et al. 1983; Barnes et al. 1985; Durelli et al. 1986; Ellison 1990; Milligan et al. 1987; Trotter and Garvey 1980) have conclusively demonstrated that administration of high-dose intravenous methylprednisolone was more effective than placebo or ACTH in producing clinical improvement from MS exacerbations. The usual regimen is 1 g methylprednisolone iv in 500 mg dextrose and water over 4 hours daily for 4 days. In our practice, we follow the intravenous therapy with oral prednisone in doses of 100 mg tapering to zero over 2 weeks, as recommended by Durelli et al. (1986). Surprisingly, side effects are usually as mild as with ACTH or a short-course oral prednisone. Gastric irritation is usually prevented by H_2-blockers or gastric mucosal barrier (Carafate), which are also routinely given.

Methylprednisolone treatment has been demonstrated to significantly improve neurological function and shorten recovery time following exacerbations (Troiano et al. 1990). Like ACTH and prednisone, it dramatically decreases IgG synthesis with the blood-brain barrier and causes a decrease of peripheral blood lymphocytes (Durelli et al. 1986). This treatment therapy may also promote resolution of CT contrast-enhancing lesions in some patients (Troiano et al. 1984) (Figure 5–2). In exacerbating disease, we reserve the methylprednisolone regimen for patients with major exacerbations that have not responded well to ACTH, or exacerbations producing major motor disability (e.g., dense paraparesis and hemiparesis).

Conventional Therapies: Chronic Progressive MS

The treatment approach for patients with chronic progressive MS differs from that for patients with exacerbating disease. The course of progressive MS is usually more predictably downhill than exacerbating disease; this permits more reliable prognostication. Remissions rarely occur and within 2 years after the onset of the chronic progressive phase, most patients will have a major disability with walking. Within 10 years after onset of chronic progression, most patients will have a relatively complete disability from the standpoint of meaningful motor function (Silberberg 1977). Treatment of chronic progressive MS must therefore be more aggressive than in exacerbating disease and delivered on as continuous a basis as possible while the disease is active.

Active chronic progressive MS is usually treated by relatively intense immunosuppression with high-dose intermittent intravenous methylprednisolone, cyclophosphamide, azathioprine, or

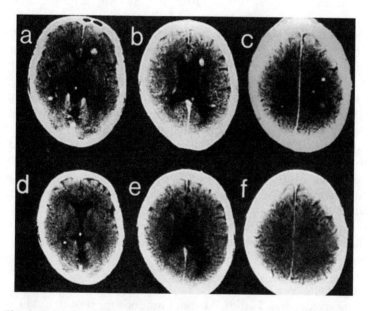

Figure 5–2. Cerebral computed tomography images with intravenous contrast of patient with multiple sclerosis before (*a*, *b*, and *c*) and after (*d*, *e*, and *f*) intravenous administration of high-dose methylprednisolone. Before methylprednisolone, there were multiple contrast-enhancing parenchymal lesions (bright), which disappeared almost completely when the study was repeated after treatment.
Source. From Troiano R, Hafstein M, Ruderman M, et al: "Effect of High-Dose Steroid Administration on Contrast-Enhancing Computed Tomographic Scan Lesions in Multiple Sclerosis." *Annals of Neurology* 15:257–263, 1984. Used with permission.

total lymphoid irradiation. Each of these therapies is associated with a variety of complications, some of which could be life-threatening. Each of the therapies is also associated with a small increase in risk for developing malignancies and opportunistic infections. Despite such significant side effects, the poor prognosis without treatment in chronic progressive MS usually warrants serious consideration of one of these agents.

Intermittent intravenous methylprednisolone. The most frequently used therapy in active chronic progressive MS is intermittent intravenous corticosteroid therapy. Although regimens vary considerably, this treatment is usually given as monthly single doses of 1–2 g methylprednisolone iv or equivalent doses of dexamethasone. The side effects of chronic corticosteroid therapy are often avoided entirely or much reduced. The therapy is continued for about 6 months, during which the patient receives one intravenous treatment (over 2–4 hours) per month. Disease activity measured clinically by monthly neurological and functional assessments is monitored. If disease activity in terms of clinical progression is halted, the treatments are discontinued. However, if the disease activity continues and clinical disability progresses, more potent immunosuppressive agents (e.g., cyclophosphamide) may be considered. Though administering intermittent intravenous corticosteroids is becoming a more generally accepted form of therapy, no prospective trials have established with certainty the benefit of this approach for chronic progressive MS.

Cyclophosphamide. Cyclophosphamide (Cytoxan), probably the most extensively studied major immunosuppressant in MS, is an alkylating agent that suppresses all leukocyte (myeloid, B cell, and T cell) immune function. Administration protocols differ from center to center. In our center, cyclophosphamide is administered in four divided daily doses of 125 mg iv in 500 ml dextrose and water for a total daily dose of 500 mg. ACTH is given simultaneously for 10 days. Metoclopramide hydrochloride (Reglan) 10 mg po or iv qid is also given as needed to decrease the nausea associated with this treatment. Therapy is continued until total white blood cell counts reach 4,000 cells/mm^3 and then is discontinued. This usually takes about 2 weeks, and, because at nadir the white blood cell counts may fall below 1,000 cells/mm^3, caution against infections must be taken. There appears to be a correlation between the degree of leukopenia achieved and the clinical benefit of the treatment. The therapy is generally well tolerated; common side effects are anorexia, nausea, and alopecia. Rarely, bone marrow suppression or chemical hepatitis (which may be life-threatening) occurs as an idiosyncratic effect. With high-dose intravenous therapy, hemorrhagic cystitis can occur. This complication is of particular concern in MS patients who may have incomplete bladder emptying and thus retain cyclophosphamide metabolites. We have found that administration of mesna simultaneously with cyclophosphamide reduces the incidence of this potentially serious complication. Bladder carcinoma, leukemia, and lymphomas have been reported following cyclophosphamide. Gonadal dysfunction and potential teratogenesis are also important considerations when using this agent.

In a study of 58 patients with chronic progressive MS, Hauser et al. (1983) found that when cyclophosphamide was administered with ACTH the benefits were superior to those found when ACTH or plasmapheresis was used alone. Eighty percent of the patients who received cyclophosphamide were stabilized after 1 year, compared to only 20% of the patients who received only ACTH and 50% of those who received plasma exchange. The favorable result of the cyclophosphamide group, compared with the ACTH group, was significant at 6 months ($P < .002$) and at 12 months ($P < .0004$). The combination of cyclophosphamide and ACTH was better than plasma exchange alone at 6 months but not at 12 months.

The beneficial effect of the cyclophosphamide lasts about 1 year, after which in most patients the disease begins to progress again (Ellison 1990). Goodkin et al. (1987) showed that by giving a maintenance therapy sufficient to lower the white blood cell count below 4,000 cells/mm^3, the favorable benefit of cyclophosphamide could be extended for 2 years. The experience with this maintenance regimen is small but potentially very important.

Currently, we use cyclophosphamide in patients who show progressive clinical deterioration despite receiving intermittent intravenous methylprednisolone or other corticosteroid therapy. Patients who are progressing to the point that walking is severely impaired and further deterioration would render them wheelchair bound are most seriously considered. Among patients already bound to a wheelchair, cyclophosphamide therapy may be used for those in whom preserved upper-extremity functions become threatened. In all cases, the risks and realistic benefits need to be discussed in detail with patients before beginning this therapy.

Azathioprine. Azathioprine (Imuran), a purine antimetabolite, is a suppressant of cellular (T-cell) more than humoral (B-cell) immune functions. Administered as a single oral dose daily, azathioprine is generally well tolerated when slowly increased to therapeutic levels. Major side effects include nausea, idiosyncratic hepatitis, and bone marrow suppression including leukopenia, thrombocytopenia, and anemia. These side effects may be delayed for several weeks after initiation of therapy.

The results of multiple trials using this substance in MS patients have been mixed (for a review, see Ellison 1990). Patzold et al. (1982) found that azathioprine 2 mg/kg body weight per day reduced the progression of disability in chronic progressive MS by about 50% when compared with control subjects after 1 year. However, Zeeberg et al. (1986) and Ellison et al. (1988) found no identifiable benefit clearly attributable to azathioprine.

The overall efficacy of azathioprine in chronic progressive disease has been difficult to assess because many patients have been unable to tolerate the drug in the doses considered to be therapeutic. Assessment of this therapy has also been difficult because of the mixed results of different investigators, sometimes assessing small numbers of patients for variable periods of follow-up and using different clinical measurements of disease progression. However, the predominance of evidence is that azathioprine slows the progression of clinical disability in chronic progressive MS. Currently, we use azathioprine in patients with chronic progressive MS who do not respond to intermittent corticosteroids and, for one reason or another, are not candidates for cyclophosphamide.

Total lymphoid irradiation. Total lymphoid irradiation may produce a long-term immunosuppression without some of the undesirable side effects or toxicities of the cytotoxic drugs described above. Such treatment administered to 45 patients with chronic progressive disease, in a dose of 1,980 rads over 45 days, resulted in a significant slowing ($P < .01$) of progression of neurological deterioration when compared with sham irradiation (Cook et al. 1987). The treatments were generally well tolerated, and it was subsequently shown that sustained neurological benefit correlated with a mean reduction in absolute lymphocyte count to less than 900 cells/mm^3. Patients who achieved this degree of lymphopenia were significantly better at 6, 12, 18, and 24 months after treatment than were those whose lymphocyte counts were greater than 900 cells/mm^3. Thus, as with cyclophosphamide and azathioprine, it seems that a critical factor determining clinical response is the reduction of leukocyte, in particular lymphocyte, counts achieved by the irradiation. The posttreatment incidence of neoplasia and opportunistic infections is currently unknown. Total lymphoid irradiation is performed at only a handful of research centers and is considered nonstandard therapy.

Experimental Therapies for MS

Interferon. A more rational immunomodulatory approach to exacerbations is the use of interferons (IFNs): naturally occurring glycoproteins produced by the human body in response to viral challenges and certain other mitogens. IFNs have marked antiviral and immunomodulatory activities. There are three types of IFNs: IFN-α, IFN-β, and IFN-γ. IFN-α and IFN-β are similar in structure and function and are referred to as *type I IFNs*. IFN-γ, referred to as *type II IFN*, has a different structure and is a more potent lymphokine than the other two.

Panitch et al. (1987) tried administering intramuscular IFN-γ to 18 exacerbating MS patients and showed that this treatment dramatically increased exacerbation rate. Immunological effects of IFN-γ treatment included increased 1) peripheral blood leukocyte proliferation, 2) number of human leukocyte antigen (HLA)-DR–bearing monocytes, and 3) natural killer cell activity. Thus treatment with IFN-γ increased both clinical exacerbations and cellular immunity, as well as disease activity within the CNS. These observations strongly suggest that MS exacerbations were being mediated by immune activation.

Unlike IFN-γ, IFN-β has been shown to reduce MS exacerbations. Moreover, in an early, small follow-up study (Jacobs et al. 1985), the reduction in exacerbation rate persisted for up to 5 years after completion of intrathecal treatment. In a larger, double-blind, placebo-controlled study of 69 exacerbating MS patients, Jacobs et al. (1986, 1987) demonstrated a significant reduction in exacerbation rate for 2 years in patients who received intrathecal IFN administered in 9–10 doses over 6 months (Figure 5–3). Thus treatment with intrathecal IFN-β resulted in a relative prophylaxis against exacerbations. The rationale for administering IFN-β intrathecally in these early studies was the belief that systemically administered IFN did not cross the blood-brain barrier (it was not found in the CSF after systemic administration). It was subsequently shown that IFN-β administered systemically did exert a direct immunological effect on CNS cells, despite its absence from the CSF (Smith et al. 1986). This latter finding made systemic administration of IFN in MS more reasonable than before.

The immunological basis for the clinical observation that IFN-β reduces exacerbations has recently become more clear (Barna et al. 1989; Ling et al. 1985). One important discovery was that IFN-γ induced HLA-DR expression on cultured human astrocytes, whereas IFN-β inhibited that expression. Astrocytes may function as antigen-presenting cells that are required for the immune response against a major histocompatibility complex (MHC)-II antigen to be activated in the CNS. This antigen may then be recognized by sensitized lymphocytes, initiating the immune response leading to inflammation and clinical exacerbation. In this fashion, the induction of HLA-DR antigen by IFN-γ may activate the immune response within the CNS causing clinical exacerbation, and IFN-β may inhibit that induction and thus prevent exacerbation.

As outlined above, MS patients may have an abnormality in suppression of the immune response leading to inflammation. Impaired immune suppressor function has been demonstrated in peripheral blood lymphocytes of MS patients (Morimoto et al. 1982; Paty et al. 1983). In a recent in vitro study, Noronha et al. (1990) showed that this impaired suppressor function of MS peripheral blood lymphocytes could be corrected by treatment with IFN-β. Thus the rationale for administering IFN-β in MS is found in the experimental evidence showing that IFN-β inhibits the expression of HLA-DR antigen on cultured astrocytes and in vitro corrects the peripheral blood suppressor-cell defect seen in MS. These phenomena (increased HLA-DR expression on astro-

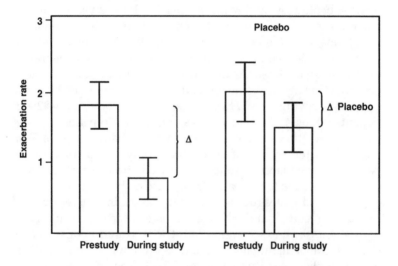

Figure 5–3. Mean exacerbation rates noted prestudy and during study in patients who received interferon-β (IFN-β) or placebo. Mean prestudy rates of both groups were nearly identical (IFN-β patients, 1.79; placebo patients, 1.98). Exacerbation rate during study of patients who received IFN-β (0.76 per year) was significantly less than that of control subjects who received placebo (1.48 per year) ($P < .001$). Changes (Δ) in exacerbation rate (i.e., decrease) of those who received IFN-β during study (1.02) were significantly greater than that of control patients (0.51) ($P < .04$). Ranges are 2 standard errors. *Source.* From Jacobs L, Salazar AM, Herndon R, et al: "Intrathecally Administered Natural Human Fibroblast Interferon Reduces Exacerbations of Multiple Sclerosis: Results of a Multicenter, Double-Blind Study." *Archives of Neurology* 44:589–595, 1987. Used with permission.

cytes and decreased peripheral blood suppressor-cell function), which may be integral parts of the MS exacerbation-remission cycle, are significantly affected by IFN-β (Salazar et al. 1983).

The clinical and laboratory studies cited above established the need for large, blind clinical studies to determine definitively the efficacy of IFN-β in treating exacerbating MS. Currently, Johnson et al. (1990) are studying 330 patients with exacerbating MS in a double-blind, multicenter trial in which patients receive either a high dose (45×10^6 units [MU]) or a low dose (9 MU) of a serine-substituted recombinant IFN-β (betaseron) or placebo administered subcutaneously three times per week for 2 years. The primary measure of this currently ongoing study is exacerbation rate. Johnson et al. reported results of a 1990 pilot study designed to examine the tolerance of this recombinant IFN-β preparation over a range of doses. A dose-related decrease in exacerbations occurred during escalation; exacerbations occurred in 40% of the patients receiving 4.5 MU three times per week but in only 22% of patients taking 45 MU three times per week. No patients taking 90 MU three times per week had an exacerbation (Figure 5–4). Similarly, after 3 years of observation, only 1 of 6 (16%) of the patients in the placebo group was exacerbation free, whereas 10 of 24 (47%) of the IFN-β patients were exacerbation free.

Jacobs and colleagues are currently assessing the efficacy of low-dose recombinant IFN-β administered intramuscularly in 312 patients with exacerbating MS. The IFN used in this study is derived from a mammalian cell line, is glycosylated, and is otherwise a replica of natural human IFN-β. The IFN used in the Johnson et al. study (1990) is derived from bacteria, is not glycosylated, has serine additions, and is therefore dissimilar from the naturally occurring human substance. As part of their ongoing study, Jacobs and colleagues have conducted a pilot study that indicated that the optimum dosage was 6 MU administered once per week over 2 years. At that dosage, IFN-β significantly induced serum microglobulin, an indirect marker of IFN biological activity, for 5 to 7 days. The pilot study also demonstrated that this was the highest dosage that could be administered under double-blind conditions.

A further difference between these studies is the primary outcome measure: exacerbation rate (Johnson) versus disability (Ja-

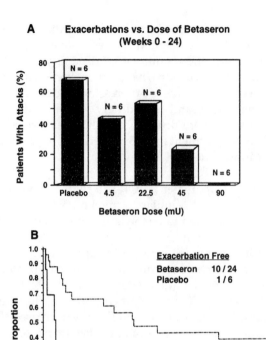

Figure 5–4. *Panel A:* Exacerbations decrease with increasing doses of a serine-substituted recombinant interferon-β (betaseron) until there were no exacerbations at highest dose. There were 6 patients treated in each group for 6 months: the number of patients with exacerbations were 4 of 6, with placebo; 3 of 7, at 4.5×10^6 units (MU) betaseron; 3 of 6, at 22.5 MU betaseron; 2 of 10, at 45 MU betaseron; and 0 of 6, at 90 MU betaseron. *Panel B:* Proportion of patients who had no exacerbations was greater in betaseron recipients than in placebo-treated patients over 6 months. At 3 years, 1 placebo-treated patient (17%) had had no exacerbations, whereas 10 betaseron patients had been free of attacks. *Source.* From Johnson KP, Knobler RL, Greenstein JI, et al: "Recombinant Human Beta Interferon Treatment of Relapsing-Remitting Multiple Sclerosis." *Neurology* 40 (suppl 1):261, 1990. Used with permission.

cobs). Disability may be the best measure of MS disease activity for several reasons. A subset of MS patients have frequent exacerbations but do not show cumulative disability and therefore, despite frequent exacerbations, have a more benign disease. Conversely, some patients have a progression in disability without definite exacerbations and accordingly, despite infrequent exacerbations, have severe disease. The entire experience to date using the IFNs as treatment for MS has recently been reviewed by Jacobs and Munschauer (1992).

Copolymer I.   Copolymer I (COP-I), a synthetic polymer polypeptide, is antigenically similar to myelin basic protein, which has long been postulated to be the target antigen of the immune attack in MS. The administration of COP-I systemically might, therefore, induce immune tolerance. In support of this, COP-I has been shown to suppress experimental allergic encephalomyelitis, an experimental model of MS (Teitelbaum et al. 1971).

In a well-designed, double-blind clinical trial, Bornstein et al. (1987) demonstrated that COP-I significantly decreased ($P < .039$) the exacerbation rate in a group of patients with exacerbating MS compared with that of placebo-treated patients. Also, the number of patients exacerbation free after 2 years was significantly higher ($P < .045$) in the COP-I group than in the placebo group. The degree of worsening on quantitative neurological examination was also less in the COP-I group than in the placebo group after 2 years of follow-up. Interestingly, in the treated patients, COP-I induced autogenous production of IFN; thus the benefit observed may have been through the IFN system. Large, phase III clinical trials of COP-I are now being designed and should establish the possible role of this agent in MS.

Monoclonal antibodies and cytokines.   Monoclonal antibodies offer an exciting and potentially effective new mode of therapy in MS. Theoretically, if the specific T-cell clone, lymphocyte, or cytokine responsible for the dysimmunity of MS was known, a monoclonal antibody against it could be generated. The offending cell or cytokine could then be removed by administering the monoclonal antibody to the patient. Unfortunately, the mechanism(s) for the immune dysfunction in MS is incompletely understood. Recently, monoclonal antibodies against the T-cell receptor, interleukin-2, and IFN-γ have been shown to have beneficial effects in the experimental model of MS, experimental allergic encephalomyelitis (Carter 1989). This evidence supports the use of such agents in MS. Clinical pilot studies of monoclonal antibodies against the pan T-cell antigen CD3 are under way.

CONCLUSIONS

MS is a disease of uncertain origins, incompletely understood dysimmunity, and unpredictable outcome that affects young individuals at their peak of productivity. Basic research into its epidemiology and immunology are now beginning to unravel the mysteries of this disease.

The current approaches to therapy use immunosuppressive and anti-inflammatory agents. The extent of immunosuppression must be tailored according to disease type and severity. In relapsing MS, ACTH is of proven value and is the agent of choice for acute exacerbations. Methylprednisolone seems also to be an excellent therapy for exacerbations, but we have less experience with it. Neither ACTH nor methylprednisolone alters the long-term course of MS. IFN-β seems to have the greatest promise for altering the course of exacerbating MS as it seems to provide prophylaxis against future relapses. No other therapy provides such prophylaxis against exacerbations or disability.

In chronic progressive MS the results of clinical trials with azathioprine have been mixed. More consistent results have been observed with cyclophosphamide, but improvement is temporary and the potential complications are serious. Total lymphoid irradiation may be as effective as cyclophosphamide, but results are transient and seem to be related, as with cyclophosphamide, to the degree of lymphocyte reduction achieved. In the long run, new approaches must be designed to attack more specifically the MS immune defect in order to alter the course of this disease.

REFERENCES

Abbruzzese G, Gandolfo C, Loeb C: "Bolus" methylprednisolone versus ACTH in the treatment of multiple sclerosis. Ital J Neurol Sci 2:169–172, 1983

Barna BP, Chou SM, Jacobs B, et al: Interferon-B impairs induction of HLS-DR antigen expression in cultured adult human astrocytes. J Neuroimmunol 23:45–53, 1989

Barnes MP, Bateman DE, Cleland PG, et al: Intravenous methylprednisolone for multiple sclerosis in relapse. J Neurol Neurosurg Psychiatry 48:157–159, 1985

Booss J, Kim JH: Evidence for a viral etiology of multiple sclerosis, in Handbook of Multiple Sclerosis. Edited by Cook SD. New York, Marcel Dekker, 1990, pp 41–62

Bornstein MB, Miller A, Slagle S, et al: A pilot trial of COP 1 in exacerbating-remitting multiple sclerosis. N Engl J Med 317:408–414, 1987

Carter JL: Immunosuppressive treatment of multiple sclerosis. Mayo Clin Proc 64:664–669, 1989

Cook SD, Devereux C, Troiano R, et al: Total lymphoid irradiation in chronic progressive multiple sclerosis: relationship between blood lymphocytes and clinical course. Ann Neurol 22:634–638, 1987

Durelli L, Cocito D, Riccio A, et al: High dose intravenous methylprednisolone in the treatment of multiple sclerosis: clinical immunological correlations. Neurology 36:238–243, 1986

Ellison GW: Chronic progressive multiple sclerosis: steroids and immunosuppressive drugs, in Handbook of Multiple Sclerosis. Edited by Cook SD. New York, Marcel Dekker, 1990, pp 371–402

Ellison GW, Myers LW, Mickey MR, et al: Clinical experience with azathioprine: the pros. Neurology 38 (suppl 2):20–23, 1988

Gessain A, Barin F, Vernant JC, et al: Antibodies to human T-lymphocytic virus type-1 in patients with tropical spastic paraparesis. Lancet 2:407–410, 1985

Goodkin DE, Plencner S, Palmer-Saxerud J, et al: Cyclophosphamide in chronic progressive multiple sclerosis; maintenance vs. nonmaintenance therapy. Arch Neurol 44:823–827, 1987

Haase AT, Ventura P, Gibbs CJ, et al: Measles virus nucleotide sequences: detection by hybridization in situ. Science 212:672–674, 1981

Hauser SL, Dawson DM, Lehrich JK, et al: Intensive immunosuppression in progressive multiple sclerosis: a randomized, three-arm study of high-dose intravenous cyclophosphamide plasma exchange, and ACTH. N Engl J Med 308:173–180, 1983

Jacobs L, Munschauer F: Treatment of multiple sclerosis with interferons, in Treatment of Multiple Sclerosis. Edited by Rudick RA, Goodkin DE. New York, Springer-Verlag, 1992, pp 233–250

Jacobs L, O'Malley JA, Freeman A, et al: Intrathecal interferon in the treatment of multiple sclerosis: patient follow-up. Arch Neurol 42:841–847, 1985

Jacobs L, Salazar AM, Herndon R, et al: Multicenter double-blind study of effect of intrathecally administered natural human fibroblast interferon on exacerbations of multiple sclerosis. Lancet 2:1411–1413, 1986

Jacobs L, Salazar AM, Herndon R, et al: Intrathecally administered natural human fibroblast interferon reduces exacerbations of multiple sclerosis: results of a multicenter double-blind study. Arch Neurol 44:589–595, 1987

Johnson KP, Knobler RL, Greenstein JI, et al: Recombinant human beta interferon treatment of relapsing-remitting multiple sclerosis (abstract). Neurology 40 (suppl 1):261, 1990

Kabat EA, Moore DH, Landow H: An electrophoretic study of the protein components in cerebrospinal fluid and their relationship to serum proteins. J Clin Invest 21:571–577, 1942

Kastrukoff KF, Oger J, Paty DW: Multiple sclerosis (MS): correlation of peripheral blood lymphocyte (PBL) phenotypes and natural killer (NK) cell activity with disease activity assessed clinically and by MRI (abstract). Ann Neurol 20:164, 1986

Khoury SJ, Weiner HL, Hafler DA: Immunologic basis of multiple sclerosis, in Handbook of Multiple Sclerosis. Edited by Cook SD. New York, Marcel Dekker, 1990, pp 129–150

Kurtzke JF: The distribution of multiple sclerosis: an update with special reference to Europe and the Mediterranean region. Acta Neurol Scand 62:65–80, 1980

Kurtzke JF: Epidemiology of multiple sclerosis, in Multiple Sclerosis. Edited by Hallpike JF, Adams CWM, Tourtellotte WW. Baltimore, MD, Williams & Wilkins, 1983, pp 47–95

Kurtzke JF, Beebe GW, Norman JE: Epidemiology of multiple sclerosis in US veterans, I: race, sex, and geographic distribution. Neurology 29:1228–1235, 1979

Ling PD, Wassen MK, Vogel SN: Antagonistic effect of interferon-B on the interferon gamma induced expression of IA antigen in macrophages. J Immunol 135:1857–1863, 1985

Miller H, Newell DJ, Ridley A: Multiple sclerosis: treatment of acute exacerbations with corticotrophin (ACTH). Lancet 2:1120–1122, 1961

Milligan NM, Newcombe R, Compton DAS: A double blind controlled trial of high dose methylprednisolone in patients with multiple sclerosis, I: clinical effects. J Neurol Neurosurg Psychiatry 50:511–516, 1987

Morimoto C, Hafler DA, Weiner HL, et al: Selective loss of the suppressor-inducer T-cell subset in progressive multiple sclerosis: analysis with anti-2H4 monoclonal antibody. N Engl J Med 316:67–72, 1982

Myers LW: Treatment of multiple sclerosis with ACTH and corticosteroids, in Treatment of Multiple Sclerosis. Edited by Rudick RA, Goodkin DE. New York, Springer-Verlag, 1992, pp 135–156

Noronha A, Toscas A, Jensen MA: Interferon beta augments suppressor cell function in multiple sclerosis. Ann Neurol 27:207–210, 1990

Oger J, Kastrukoff LF, Li DKB, et al: Multiple sclerosis: in relapsing patients, immune functions vary with disease activity as assessed by MRI. Neurology 38:1739–1743, 1988

Panitch HS, Heracl RL, Schindler J, et al: Treatment of multiple sclerosis with gamma interferon: exacerbations associated with activation of the immune system. Neurology 37:1097–1102, 1987

Paty DW, Kastrukoff L, Morgan N, et al: Suppressor T-lymphocytes in multiple sclerosis: analysis of patients with acute relapsing and chronic progressive disease. Ann Neurol 14:445–449, 1983

Patzold U, Hecker H, Pocklington P, et al: Azathioprine in treatment of multiple sclerosis: final results of a 4 1/2 year controlled study of its effectiveness covering 115 patients. J Neurol Sci 54:377–394, 1982

Rice GPA, Casali P, Merigan TC, et al: Natural killer cell activity in patients with multiple sclerosis given interferon. Ann Neurol 14:333–338, 1983

Rodriguez M: Multiple sclerosis: basic concepts and hypothesis. Mayo Clin Proc 64:570–576, 1989

Rose AAS, Kuzma JW, Kurtzke JF, et al: Cooperative study in the evaluation of therapy in multiple sclerosis: ACTH vs. placebo: final report. Neurology 20 (suppl):1–59, 1970

Rudick RA, Pallant A, Bidlock JM, et al: Free kappa light chains in multiple sclerosis spinal fluid. Ann Neurol 20:63–69, 1986

Salazar AM, Gibbs CJ, Gajusek CK, et al: Clinical use of interferons: central nervous system disorders, in Handbook of Experimental Pharmacology, Vol 71. Edited by Came P, Carter WA. New York, Springer-Verlag, 1983, pp 472–497

Silberberg D: Multiple sclerosis, in Scientific Approaches to Clinical Neurology, Vol 10. Edited by Goldensohn ES, Appel SH. Philadelphia, PA, Lea & Febiger, 1977, 10:299–324

Smith RA, Landel C, Cornelius CE, et al: Mapping the action of interferon on the primate brain. J Interferon Res 6 (Suppl 1):140, 1986

Teitelbaum D, Meshorer A, Hirshfeld T, et al: Suppression of experimental allergic encephalomyelitis by a synthetic polypeptide. Eur J Immunol 1:242–248, 1971

terMeulen V, Stephenson JR: The possible role of viral infections in multiple sclerosis and other related demyelinating diseases, in Multiple Sclerosis. Edited by Hallpike JF, Adams CWM, Tourtellotte WW. Baltimore, MD, Williams & Wilkins, 1983, pp 241–274

Troiano R, Hafstein M, Ruderman M, et al: Effect of high-dose steroid administration on contrast-enhancing computed tomographic scan lesions in multiple sclerosis. Ann Neurol 15:257–263, 1984

Troiano R, Cook SD, Dowling PC: Corticosteroid therapy in acute multiple sclerosis, in Handbook of Multiple Sclerosis. Edited by Cook SD. New York, Marcel Dekker, 1990, pp 351–369

Trotter JL, Garvey WF: Prolonged effects of large-dose methylprednisolone infusion in multiple sclerosis. Neurology 30:702–708, 1980

Zeeberg I, Heltberg A, Kristensen JH, et al: A long-term, double-blind controlled trial of azathioprine versus placebo in treatment of progressive multiple sclerosis, in Immunotherapies in Multiple Sclerosis. Edited by Hommes OR, Mertin JG, Tourtellotte WW. Sutton, England, Stuart Phillips, 1986, pp 295–302

Chapter 6

Psychosomatic-Somatopsychic Aspects of Multiple Sclerosis

Igor Grant, M.D., F.R.C.P.C.

T he natural course of many medical and neurological illnesses can be influenced by psychosocial factors such as
stressful life events, quality and number of social supports, and
the nature of coping activity. Among the neurological illnesses,
multiple sclerosis (MS) has long been considered to have psycho-
somatic and somatopsychic elements (i.e., it has been speculated
that personal-environmental factors could influence the onset
and natural history of MS, and the neuropathogenic process
could alter cognition, mood, and behavior). In this chapter, I
review briefly the "psychological" correlates of MS, examine in
some detail the current state of understanding of the role of
stressful life events on onset and exacerbation of symptoms, and
conclude with a brief review of adaptational changes in MS. As
other chapters in this volume provide extensive reviews of neuropsychological and affective changes, I have kept this discussion to the minimum necessary to set a stage for understanding
the more in-depth discussion of "stress" that forms the principal
focus of this chapter.

PSYCHOLOGICAL MANIFESTATIONS IN MS

The common psychological manifestations in MS include cognitive changes (intellectual functions and memory), depression,
elation and affective lability, and fatigue. (For recent reviews in
this area, see Jensen et al. 1989; Rao 1990.)

Support for this review was provided in part by Award SA320 to I. Grant from the
Veterans Affairs Medical Research Service. The author thanks Mary Eskes for her
excellent help in the preparation of this manuscript. This work is in the public
domain.

Cognitive Changes

Cognitive disturbances were recognized in patients with MS as early as Charcot's first clinical descriptions of the entity (1877). It is currently thought that, tested by suitable neuropsychological means, approximately half of an unselected group of patients with MS will manifest some neuropsychological deficit (Grant 1986; Grant et al. 1989a; Jouvent et al. 1989; Rao 1990; Trimble and Grant 1982). A range of cognitive functions can be affected, including reaction time (Jennekens-Schinkel et al. 1988), early information processing (Rao et al. 1989a), various aspects of memory (Grant et al. 1984; Rao et al. 1989b), complex perceptual motor abilities (Filley et al. 1989; Grant et al. 1984), and abstracting ability (for reviews, see Grant 1986; Trimble and Grant 1982).

Cognitive deficits can present very early in the course of MS, during a time when patients may be essentially asymptomatic from a gross neurological standpoint. For example, Grant et al. (1984, 1989a) noted that defects in learning and recall were seen in patients ill for less than 5 years, whereas Jouvent et al. (1989) found that 46% of 37 patients with either optic neuritis or MS for less than 2 years had some cognitive defect. In general, degree of cognitive impairment is related to later disease stage (e.g., years of disease or disability status as measured by the Kurtzke Extended Disability Status Scale [Kurtzke 1983]) (Grant 1986; Grant et al. 1989a; Petersen and Kokmen 1989), although some investigators (e.g., Iwasaki et al. 1989) have not agreed that such a correlation to functional abilities exists.

Cognitive impairment also appears to relate to amount and location of cerebral lesions as identified through magnetic resonance imaging (MRI). Patients with extensive periventricular demyelination are thought to be especially likely to have cognitive deficits (Anzola et al. 1990; Reischies et al. 1988). However, even patients with seemingly "clinically isolated" lesions can show performance deficit (Callanan et al. 1989). Occasionally, cognitive changes may be the first or primary symptoms heralding the onset of MS (Felgenhauer 1990). At present, it is not clear whether a relapsing-remitting or a chronic progressive clinical picture is related to differing likelihood of cognitive disturbance (Beatty et al. 1990).

Depression

Depression is the most common mood disturbance experienced by patients with MS. The point prevalence has been estimated to range from 27% to 54% (Minden and Schiffer 1990), although rates as low as 6% have been estimated (Kahana et al. 1971). Both the point prevalence and lifetime prevalence (42% in Joffe et al. 1987; 54% in Minden et al. 1987) exceed most estimates for mood disorder in medical patients in the general population and in patients with other neurological diseases, such as amyotrophic lateral sclerosis (Minden and Schiffer 1990).

In attempting to understand the causation of depressive disorder associated with MS, Berrios and Quemada (1990) proposed three possibilities: coincidence, reactivity, and organic causation. Coincidence is unlikely given the preponderance of evidence showing very substantially increased point and lifetime prevalence of mood disorder in patients with MS. Reactivity (i.e., depression as "response" to a serious illness) probably accounts for depression in some MS patients, but this mechanism cannot be fully explanatory given contradictory reports concerning association (and lack thereof) between severity of MS symptomatology, degree of disability, and length of illness and likelihood to experience mood disorder (Berrios and Quemada 1990).

That at least part of the depression is explained by neurobiological processes is made plausible by several observations that suggest that the extent and location of lesions of demyelination, as imaged by MRI, relate to the likelihood of mood disturbance. For example, extent of periventricular lesions was linked to mood disturbance by Reischies et al. (1988), and observations by Honer et al. (1987) and Rabins et al. (1986) indicate that patients with a greater preponderance of "central" lesions were more likely to experience depression. Periodic observations that depressive symptoms can precede and herald the onset of MS lend credence to the organic hypothesis as well (Minden and Schiffer 1990).

In reality, the increased prevalence of depression in MS probably cannot be explained solely either by organic or reactivity theories or even by a combination of these. Rather, it seems more likely that such an understanding emerges better from full recourse to the "psychosomatic-somatopsychic" frame of reference. Such a point of view would predict that

1. People with cerebral disease, particularly in areas of the brain involved in modulation of affect (limbic lobe and intimately connected structures) are more likely to experience mood disorders. In this sense, the demyelinating process "causes" depression.
2. People experiencing major illnesses of unknown etiology, uncertain natural history, and lacking effective treatment are naturally more likely to become depressed.
3. People with MS also appear to be at heightened risk to experience adverse life events, and such major life stresses have been associated with onsets and exacerbation of depression in other subject groups (for reviews, see Brown and Harris 1989). Indeed, Ron and Logsdail (1989) found that dysphoric symptoms in their sample of MS patients were highest in those who experienced more life events of various sorts.
4. People with neurocognitive disturbance may be more vulnerable to experiencing depression by virtue of compromised range and flexibility of coping. If this were true, mood and cognitive disturbance would not occur in parallel. For example, in early MS there could be more depression, yet slight cognitive impairment; however, as cognitive capacities became more severely impaired, depressive reaction would become less likely. This is because a refined evaluation of the meaning of a person's circumstance would become less possible. Therefore, people with more severe cognitive breakdown should experience less depression, which is actually what is observed (Berrios and Quemada 1990; Minden and Schiffer 1990).

Elation and Lability of Affect

Inappropriately exhilarated affect, coupled with an abnormal sense of well-being, has long been observed in some persons with advanced MS. Some of the best descriptions of these phenomena come from Cottrell and Wilson's series (1926) in which they considered that euphoria and eutonia (an unusual sense of physical well-being) were characteristic symptoms of MS. After reviewing the literature, Minden and Schiffer (1990) concluded that euphoria can be regarded as an abnormal neurologically based emotional state that occurs primarily with advanced disseminated cerebral demyelination. The exact prevalence is not known, with a range of 6%–63% being reported in various series (see, Minden and Schiffer 1990). The current understanding, however, is that euphoria and lability (pathological laughing and weeping) occur principally in advanced disease and that the prevalence is about 10% (Minden and Schiffer 1990).

The euphoria of MS is not identical to the elation seen in bipolar disorders. Although there may be a sense of well-being, it is generally not accompanied by accelerated thinking, push of speech, flight of ideas, and grandiose delusions. Etiologically, euphoria has been linked to more advanced cerebral demyelination, coupled with cognitive decline. Both euphoria and affective lability may be products of progressive disconnection between limbic structures that generate affect and cortical regions responsible for evaluation of self and environment.

Fatigue

Fatigue is perhaps the most common subjective complaint of patients with MS. Often it is the first reported symptom before diagnosis; it is also among the most troublesome symptoms that MS patients experience (Krupp et al. 1988). *Fatigue* has been defined as a sense of tiredness or lack of energy greater than expected for the degree of effort required for a task or degree of disability (Canadian Research Group 1987). This sense of tiredness and lack of energy is distinct from sadness or weakness (Krupp et al. 1988). Symptoms of fatigue increase as the day goes on (Cohen and Fisher 1989) but do not appear to be related to severity of physical disability produced by MS (Krupp et al. 1988).

Fatigue is a distinct symptom complex in MS; that is, despite sharing some superficial features with depressed mood (which can also be accompanied by a sense of fatigue and lack of motivation), the fatigue state in MS does not appear to be linked to depression. For example, correlations between subjective ratings of fatigue and depressive symptoms tend to be low (Krupp et al. 1988), and traditional antidepressants do not confer striking benefits. Although fatigue in MS has qualitative similarities to the fatigue experienced by healthy people, the prevalence of moderate-to-severe fatigue is substantially higher in MS (65% versus 15% [Krupp et al. 1988]). Furthermore, MS patients are more likely to report that their fatigue is worsened by heat, comes on easily, and interferes significantly with their ability to meet daily obligations (Krupp et al. 1988). Amantadine, an antiparkinsonian agent with dopamine-releasing properties, has been reported as variably effective in improving some aspects of MS-related fatigue (Cohen and Fisher 1989; Canadian Research Group 1987). From the psychosomatic-somatopsychic point of view, the phenomenon of fatigue is important to acknowledge because it constitutes yet another factor that may influence the ability of a person with MS to adapt flexibly both to life stresses and progression of disease.

LIFE STRESSES IN RELATION TO ONSET AND EXACERBATION OF MS

Although the first pathological description of MS has been attributed to Sir Robert Carswell of University College, London, the first recorded case study appears in the autobiographical notes of Augustus d'Este, illegitimate son of Prince Augustus Frederick, sixth son of King George III of England (transcribed by Firth [1948]).

It is interesting that in this first case description, there are immediate suggestions of an association between "stress" and onset of clinical symptoms of MS. D'Este wrote the following account of a trip to Scotland where he expected to spend some time with a relative . . .

> for whom I had the affection of Son. On my arrival I found him dead. I attended his funeral: -there being many persons present I struggled *violently not to weep*, I was however, unable to prevent myself from so doing: - Shortly after the funeral I was obliged to have my letters read to me, and their answers written for me, as my eyes were so attacked that when fixed upon minute objects

indistinctness of vision was the consequence: - Until I attempted to read, or to cut my pen, I was not aware of my Eyes being in the least attacked. Soon after, I went to Ireland, and without anything having been done to my Eyes, they completely recovered their strength and distinctness of vision. (Firth 1948, p. 25)

The next episode of optic neuritis appears once more to coincide with a stressful period in d'Este's life. His mother had been seriously ill in Paris, and his courtship of a Princess Feodora of Leiningen had been forcibly terminated by his outraged father. D'Este wrote

In the month of January, 1826, the most painful Chapter up to that period of my life occurred, I was beset by afflictions on all sides. My Eyes were again attacked in the same manner as they had been in Scotland (Firth 1948, p. 25).

Early clinical accounts also alluded to the possible role of life circumstances in progression of MS. For example, Charcot (1877), who provided the first accurate clinical description of MS, noted in an 1868 lecture at la Salpêtrière, "But the circumstances most commonly assigned as causes of this disease, by patients have pertained to the moral order—long continued grief or vexation" (p. 220). The English neurologist Moxon (1873) also described a case in which onset of MS symptoms seemed to relate to a severe life stress. He wrote, "Aetiologically it is important to mention another statement the poor creature made when giving a more confidential account to the nurse—vis., that the cause of her disease was having caught her husband in bed with another woman. It was not possible to learn how far this was right; but she was neglected by her friends" (p. 236).

In the 1940s and 50s, there were a number of case observations and uncontrolled series that provided speculative associations, often from a psychoanalytic perspective, between stressful life circumstances and symptomatology in MS. Langworthy et al. (1941) reported that female patients with MS were emotionally immature; were caught in entangling neurotic relationships with their mothers, seeking independence through marriage, but in so doing married "losers"; and attributed onset of illness to circumstances when conflict between submission and dominance was reactivated, for example, if the "loser" husband were actually to "succeed" ultimately (Langworthy 1948, 1950; Langworthy et al. 1941).

Grinker et al. (1950) conducted psychoanalytic interviews with 20 men and 6 women with MS. They observed that life events stimulating "intense resentment or anger" appeared to precede onset. Brickner and Simons (1950) performed record reviews of 50 patients with MS. They noted that 15 of the 50 had experienced stressful life experiences. On the other hand, Braceland and Giffin (1950), who performed psychiatric interviews with 75 MS patients, concluded that psychogenic causes could be assigned not only for MS, but for any other control series as well.

In a more detailed psychoanalytic study, Philippopoulous et al. (1958) examined 22 men and 18 women with MS whose duration of illness was typically less than 5 years. After conducting detailed psychiatric interviews, they observed that, before onset of symptoms, 35 of 40 patients experienced traumatic life events that had threatened their "security system."

An interesting and in-depth psychoanalytic study was conducted by Engel's group (Mei-Tal et al. 1970), but, unfortunately, this study was also uncontrolled. The investigators performed psychoanalytically oriented interviews with 32 MS patients and observed that 28 of them had experienced a stressful situation generating the "giving up–given up" complex (i.e., sensing that he or she will fail to cope with specific challenges, the patient anticipates being disapproved of or rejected by important others; this generates an overwhelming sense of helplessness—there is a fear of "giving up" coupled with a threat of being "given up" on) before the onset of symptoms.

Controlled studies have reached more variable conclusions concerning the potential association between stressful life events and symptomatology in MS. The first of the properly controlled studies was that of Pratt (1951). He examined 50 men and 50 women with MS and matched these with 100 neurological patients with other diagnoses. He performed interviews probing for "emotional antecedents" to onset or symptom exacerbation. Pratt noted that 38% of patients with MS, versus 26% of the control subjects, had "antecedents." This difference in proportion was not statistically significant. At the same time, Pratt noted that a subset of the MS patients did appear to have symptom exacerbations in relation to major life stresses.

Antonovsky et al. (1968) conducted structured interviews with 221 patients who, on average, had had MS for more than 10 years. Interviews were conducted also with 442 healthy control subjects. Of nine areas of inquiry, "very difficult interpersonal relationships" were found to be significantly higher in MS patients (19%) than in control subjects (12%) ($P < .01$). Clearly, although this difference was statistically significant, the clinical importance of a 7% spread must be questioned.

Of the more recent studies, the largest was that reported by Warren et al. (1982). Warren and her colleagues examined 100 patients with MS and 73 neurological-rheumatological patients. Interviews revealed that, in the 2 years before onset, patients with MS had more events of all sorts than did control subjects (180 versus 59). Also, more MS patients felt "unusually stressed" during that period (79% versus 54%) and more had life events that received higher (greater than 40) readjustment ratings on Holmes and Rahe's Schedule of Recent Experiences (SRE; Holmes and Rahe 1967) (18% versus 4%).

Franklin et al. (1988) reported a follow-up of 55 patients with remitting-relapsing MS. The Psychiatric Epidemiology Research Interview (PERI; Dohrenwend et al. 1978) for life events was administered every 4 months for approximately 20 months. The results indicated that patients with significant negative or uncontrollable events in the preceding 4 months were 3.7 times more likely to suffer an exacerbation than those patients who were free of such events. These data are important in that they are among the first from a prospective study to provide a temporal association between undesirable events and exacerbations.

In a report linking affective disorder and stress in MS, Stip (1988) compared the life events scores of 35 MS patients with the scores of a comparison series of medical patients. The SRE was used again. Life events scores were significantly higher in the MS group ($P < .001$). Further, there was a significant relationship between dysphoria and the life events score ($P < .01$).

Grant et al. (1989b) performed a study with 39 patients at various stages of MS and 40 sociodemographically matched control subjects. One methodological refinement in this particular study was the use of the interview-based Life Events and Difficulties Schedule (LEDS), developed at the Bedford College of London University by Brown and Harris (1989). This approach permits a systematic guided inquiry into life circumstances in the preceding 12 months. Happenings are classified as "incidents" if they appear not to pose any obvious "threat" to life situation. The remaining happenings are classified as "events," if they involve circumstances occurring in a relatively discrete time frame, or as "difficulties" if they stretch beyond a month. More importantly, the LEDS system permits "contextual" rating of the threat, focus of events, and independence by the *investigators* working in a case conference mode. Such contextual ratings can serve to dampen variations occasioned by idiosyncratic amplification or denial of the seriousness of events in self-report data.

In the LEDS, the threat of an event is rated on a 4-point scale: 1 = very severe, 2 = moderate to severe, 3 = mild to moderate, and 4 = minimal threat. Events are rated in terms of focus, with a "self-focus" rating signifying happenings that occur directly to the individual in question or directly involve the individual in some manner. An "other-focus" rating is reserved for events that occur to other individuals. Such events need not be unimportant; but they do not *directly* involve the index person as an actor in the circumstance. For example, the death of a beloved aunt in Australia is rated as other-focused if the patient lives in Canada. The death of a beloved aunt may be rated as self-focused if the aunt resided in the same city as the patient and the patient was actually involved in caring for the aunt or making the funeral arrangements. Finally, it is possible to rate events in terms of "independence," in which case events that may be "caused" by the disease itself should be taken out of any analysis in which events are hypothesized to be provoking agents. For example, a patient has an automobile accident, a rather stressful event. If, however, the accident is related to visual problems or psychomotor difficulties that are part of MS, it would be classed as a "dependent" event.

Difficulties are circumstances that continue for more than 1 month. These are also rated on a severity scale, that ranges from 1 = extremely severe to 6 = very mild. Contextual ratings of this sort permit an additional summary classification of life circumstances, which involves deciding whether a patient has experienced a "marked life adversity" in the time frame of interest. A marked life adversity is said to exist if a patient experienced 1) a level-1 threatening event, no matter what the focus; 2) a level-2 threatening event with a self-focus; 3) a difficulty with a level-1, -2, or -3 threatening event; or 4) any combination of the above.

Based on such a rating scheme, Grant et al. (1989b) found that 30 of 39 MS patients (77%) reported marked life adversity in the 12 months preceding onset of their symptomatology. In contrast, 14 of 40 (35%) nonpatient control subjects experienced marked adversity in a 12-month period. More detailed examination of the data revealed that threatening life events (i.e., level-1 threatening events with either self- or other-focus, or level-2 threatening events with a self-focus) increased substantially in the 6 months before onset in MS patients (compared with months 7–12), but other more trivial events did not show such a marked rise (Figures 6–1 and 6–2). These data are among the first to show that *specific* life circumstances of a highly threatening nature were associated to MS onset or exacerbation, as opposed to accumulation of "little events" or "hassles." The most common classes of

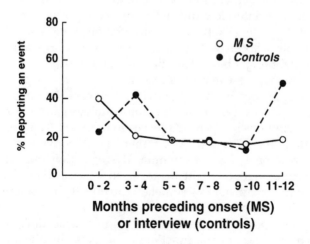

Figure 6–1. Report of severely threatening life events by 39 patients with multiple sclerosis (MS) and 40 control subjects.

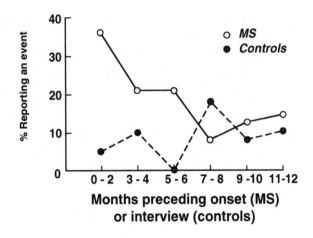

Figure 6–2. Report of less threatening events by 39 patients with multiple sclerosis (MS) and 40 control subjects.

adversity were conflicts or prolonged separations involving a spouse, close family member, or other confiding person; major illness or death of a loved one or "confidant"; major work-related problems; major interpersonal conflicts; and housing problems. Interestingly, whether or not a patient knew his or her diagnosis at the time of interview did not influence reporting of events, which makes it less likely that "effort after meaning" encouraged the patients who knew they had MS to overreport events that they thought might be contributing to their illness.

In summary, research on stressful life events has produced mixed results, but most of the evidence favors the notion that both onset and exacerbation of symptomatology can be linked to major disruptions in a person's social environment. This does not mean that stress "causes" MS; rather, the underlying process, which presumably involves immune dysregulation and perhaps an infectious agent, might be revealed or exacerbated when stressful life circumstances somehow disrupt the neuroimmune system. One important challenge facing future investigators is to define more precisely whether changes in neuroendocrine factors, lymphokines, or the functioning of the sympathoadrenal-medullary system can somehow contribute to progress of the immunoneuropathogenic process.

ADAPTATION IN MS

Despite the fact that MS can bring with it problematic and disabling symptoms, that there are no truly effective treatments, and that patients recognize that their prognosis may ultimately be unfavorable, many adjust remarkably well to their condition. Zeldow and Pavlou (1988) recently reported on a cluster analytic study with 81 patients who were administered the California Psychological Inventory (CPI; Gough 1969) and the Sickness Impact Profile (SIP; Gilson et al. 1985). The authors noted that 44% of their patients had good adjustments, essentially indistinguishable from patterns found among nonpatient control subjects. A smaller fraction (12%) were people who were clearly unhappy and frustrated by their illness, yet behaved in a highly self-reliant manner. The remaining patients had more dysfunctional adaptive styles. For example, 22% exhibited euphoric mood, psychosocial deficit, and an absence of self-awareness, whereas another 21% appeared to behave in a more outgoing, overbearing, and self-centered manner. Patients in the last cluster also experienced more life events based on the SRE. Although such descriptive clusters have obvious limitations, what the data do demonstrate is that approximately half of patients with MS are coping very well indeed.

One important determinant of better adaptation appears to be the quality of the social support network the MS patient has. Wineman (1990) noted that depression in her sample was related to perceived unsupportiveness of the social net. An unsupportive environment was also found to be correlated with "reduced purpose in life."

These data are consistent with earlier reports that better psychological adaptation in MS is associated with better perceived social support (McIvor et al. 1984; Pollock et al. 1990), propinquity to a significant other (Miles 1979), and more frequent opportunity to interact with physically healthy people (Maybury and Brewin 1984). Indeed, data on the importance of social support to psychological adaptation in MS tend to be more consistent than the data on attempts to relate depressed mood to functional disability and length of illness. Here, although some investigators found depression to be linked to degree of handicap and length of illness (e.g., McIvor et al. 1984; Whitlock and Siskind 1980), others have not observed such a relationship (Minden et al. 1987; Rabins et al. 1986).

SUMMARY

From this review it can be seen that much still needs to be learned about adaptational processes in MS. In particular, future research will need to consider biological factors (e.g, nature of neurological symptoms, their duration, and their periodicity) and psychological phenomena (e.g., depressed mood, fatigue, and cognitive inefficiency) in the context of the patient's broader life circumstances. The latter will require the assessment of stressful life events (marked adversities) and the extent and quality of supportive relationships. Such biological and psychosocial data will then need to be linked to more sophisticated assessments of coping activity, made possible with instruments such as the Ways of Coping (Folkman and Lazarus 1988).

In attempting to develop actual causal models, it will be important to expand the biological assessments to include measures of neuroendocrine and immune functioning. If there are connections among stress, mood, coping, and disease progression, such biological variables (neuroendocrines and lymphokines) may serve as mediating links in such a relationship. In this manner, we may come closer to understanding the real nature of MS as a psychosomatic-somatopsychic disease process.

REFERENCES

Antonovsky A, Leibowitz U, Medalle JM, et al: Reappraisal of possible etiologic factors in multiple sclerosis. Am J Public Health 58:836–848, 1968

Anzola GP, Bevilacqua L, Cappa SF, et al: Neuropsychological assessment in patients with relapsing-remitting multiple sclerosis and mild functional impairment: correlation with magnetic resonance imaging. J Neurol Neurosurg Psychiatry 53:142–145, 1990

Beatty WW, Goodkin DE, Hertsgaard D, et al: Clinical and demographic predictors of cognitive performance in multiple sclerosis: do diagnostic type, disease duration, and disability matter? Arch Neurol 47:305–308, 1990

Berrios GE, Quemada JI: Depressive illness in MS: clinical and theoretical aspects of the association. Br J Psychiatry 156:10–16, 1990

Braceland FJ, Giffin ME: The mental changes associated with multiple sclerosis: an interim report. Proceedings of the Association for Research in Nervous and Mental Diseases 28:450–455, 1950

Brickner RM, Simons DJ: Emotional stress in relation to attacks of multiple sclerosis. Proceedings of the Association for Research in Nervous and Mental Diseases 28:143–145, 1950

Brown G, Harris T (eds): Life Events and Illness. London, Guilford, 1989

Callanan MM, Logsdail SJ, Ron MA, et al: Cognitive impairment in patients with clinically isolated lesions of the type seen in multiple sclerosis: a psychometric and MRI study, in Mental Disorders and Cognitive Deficits in Multiple Sclerosis. Edited by Jensen J, Knudsen L, Stenager E, et al. London, John Libbey, 1989, pp 63–75

Canadian Research Group: A randomized controlled trial of amantadine in fatigue associated with multiple sclerosis. Can J Neurol Sci 14:273–278, 1987

Charcot JM: Lectures on the Diseases of the Nervous System delivered at La Salpêtrière. London, New Sydenham Society, 1877

Cohen RA, Fisher M: Amantadine treatment of fatigue associated with multiple sclerosis. Arch Neurol 46:676–680, 1989

Cottrell SS, Wilson SK: The affective symptomatology of disseminated sclerosis. Journal of Neurology and Psychopathology 7:1–30, 1926

Dohrenwend BS, Krasnoff L, Askenagy AR, et al: Exemplification of a method for scaling life events: the PERI life events scale. J Health Soc Behav 19:205–229, 1978

Felgenhauer K: Psychiatric disorders in the encephalitic form of multiple sclerosis. J Neurol 237:11–18, 1990

Filley CM, Heaton RK, Nelson LM, et al: A comparison of dementia in Alzheimer's disease and multiple sclerosis. Arch Neurol 46:157–161, 1989

Firth D: The Case of Augustus d'Este. Cambridge, England, Cambridge University Press, 1948

Folkman S, Lazarus RS: Coping as a mediator of emotion. J Pers Soc Psychol 54:466–475, 1988

Franklin GM, Nelson LM, Heaton RK, et al: Stress and its relationship to acute exacerbations in multiple sclerosis. Journal of Neurological Rehabilitation 2:7–11, 1988

Gilson BS, Gilson JS, Bergner M, et al. The Sickness Impact Profile: development of an outcome measure of health care. Am J Publ Health 65:1304–1310, 1985

Gough HG: Manual for the California Psychological Inventory, Palo Alto, CA, Consulting Psychologists Press, 1969

Grant I: Neuropsychological and psychiatric disturbances in multiple sclerosis, in Multiple Sclerosis. Edited by McDonald WI, Silberberg DH. London, Butterworths, 1986, pp 134–152

Grant I, McDonald WI, Trimble MR, et al: Deficient learning and memory in early and middle phases of multiple sclerosis. J Neurol Neurosurg Psychiatry 57:250–255, 1984

Grant I, McDonald WI, Trimble MR: Neuropsychological impairment in early multiple sclerosis, in Mental Disorders and Cognitive Deficits in Multiple Sclerosis. Edited by Jensen K, Knudsen L, Stenager E, et al. London, John Libbey, 1989a, p 17–26

Grant I, Brown GW, Harris T, et al: Severely threatening events and marked life difficulties preceding onset or exacerbation of multiple sclerosis. J Neurol Neurosurg Psychiatry 52:8–13, 1989b

Grinker RR, Ham GV, Robbins FP: Some psychodynamic factors in multiple sclerosis. Proceedings of the Association for Research in Nervous and Mental Diseases 28:456–460, 1950

Holmes TJ, Rahe RH: The social readjustment rating scale. J Psychosom Res 11:213–218, 1967

Honer WG, Hurwitz T, Li DKB, et al: Temporal lobe involvement in multiple sclerosis patients with psychiatric disorders. Arch Neurol 44:187–190, 1987

Iwasaki Y, Kinoshita M, Ikeda K, et al: Cognitive function in multiple sclerosis and its relation to functional abilities. Int J Neurosci 48(3–4):219–223, 1989

Jennekens-Schinkel A, Sanders EA, Lanser JB, et al: Reaction time in ambulant multiple sclerosis patients, I: influence of prolonged cognitive effect. J Neurol Sci 85:175–186, 1988

Jensen K, Knudsen L, Stenager E, et al (eds): Mental Disorders and Cognitive Deficits in Multiple Sclerosis. London, John Libbey, 1989

Joffe RT, Lippert GP, Gray TA, et al: Personal and family history of affective illness in patients with multiple sclerosis. J Affective Disord 44:187–190, 1987

Jouvent R, Montreuil M, Benoit N, et al: Cognitive impairment, emotional disturbances and duration of multiple sclerosis, in Mental Disorders and Cognitive Deficits in Multiple Sclerosis. Edited by Jensen K, Knudsen L, Stenager E, et al. London, John Libbey, 1989, pp 139–145

Kahana E, Leibowitz U, Alter M: Cerebral multiple sclerosis. Neurology 21:1179–1185, 1971

Krupp LB, Alvarez LA, LaRocca NG, et al: Fatigue in multiple sclerosis. Arch Neurol 45:435–437, 1988

Kurtzke JF: Rating neurologic impairment in multiple sclerosis: an expanded disability status scale (EDSS). Neurology 33:1422–1427, 1983

Langworthy OR: Relation of personality problems to onset and progress of multiple sclerosis. Archives of Neurology and Psychiatry 59:13–28, 1948

Langworthy OR: A survey of the maladjustment problems in multiple sclerosis and the possibilities of psychotherapy. Proceedings of the Association for Research in Nervous and Mental Diseases 28:598–611, 1950

Langworthy OR, Kolb LC, Anthrop S: Disturbances of behavior in patients with disseminated sclerosis. Am J Psychiatry 98:243–249, 1941

Maybury CP, Brewin CR: Social relationships, knowledge and adjustment to multiple sclerosis. J Neurol Neurosurg Psychiatry 47:372–376, 1984

McIvor GP, Riklan M, Reznikoff M: Depression in multiple sclerosis as a function of length and severity of illness, age, remissions and perceived social support. J Clin Psychol 40:1028–1033, 1984

Mei-Tal V, Meyerowitz S, Engel GL: The role of psychological process in a somatic disorder: multiple sclerosis. Psychosom Med 32:67–86, 1970

Miles A: Some psycho-social consequences of multiple sclerosis: problems of social interaction and group identity. Br J Med Psychol 52:321–331, 1979

Minden SL, Schiffer RB: Affective disorders in multiple sclerosis: review and recommendations for clinical research. Arch Neurol 47:98–104, 1990

Minden SL, Orav J, Reich P: Depression in multiple sclerosis. Gen Hosp Psychiatry 9:426–434, 1987

Moxon W: Case of insular sclerosis of brain and spinal cord. Lancet 1:236, 1873

Petersen RC, Kokmen E: Cognitive and psychiatric abnormalities in multiple sclerosis. Mayo Clin Proc 64:657–663, 1989

Philippopoulos GS, Wittkower ED, Cousineau A: The etiologic significance of emotional factors in onset and exacerbations of multiple sclerosis. Psychosom Med 20:458–474, 1958

Pollock SE, Christian BJ, Sands D: Responses to chronic illness: analysis of psychological and physiological adaptation. Nurs Res 39:300–304, 1990

Pratt RC: An investigation of the psychiatric aspects of disseminated sclerosis. J Neurol Neurosurg Psychiatry 14:326–336, 1951

Rabins PV, Brooks BR, O'Donnell P, et al: Structural brain correlates of emotional disorder in multiple sclerosis. Brain 109:585–597, 1986

Rao SM (ed): Multiple Sclerosis: A Neuropsychological Approach. New York, Oxford University Press, 1990

Rao SM, St. Aubin-Faubert P, Leo GJ: Information processing in multiple sclerosis. J Clin Exp Neuropsychol 11:471–477, 1989a

Rao SM, Leo GJ, St. Aubin-Faubert P: On the nature of memory disturbance in multiple sclerosis. J Clin Exp Neuropsychol 11:699–712, 1989b

Reischies FM, Baum K, Brau H, et al: Cerebral magnetic resonance imaging findings in multiple sclerosis. Arch Neurol 45:1114–1116, 1988

Ron MA, Logsdail SJ: Psychiatric morbidity in multiple sclerosis: a clinical and MRI study. Psychol Med 19:887–895, 1989

Stip E: Affective disorder and stress in multiple sclerosis (letter). Psychosomatics 29:454, 1988

Trimble MR, Grant I: Psychiatric aspects of multiple sclerosis, in Psychiatric Aspects of Neurologic Disease, Vol 2. Edited by Benson DF, Blumer D. New York, Grune & Stratton, 1982, pp 279–299

Warren S, Greenhill S, Warren KG: Emotional stress and the development of multiple sclerosis: case-control evidence of a relationship. Journal of Chronic Disease 35:821–831, 1982

Whitlock FA, Siskind MM: Depression as a major symptom of multiple sclerosis. J Neurol Neurosurg Psychiatry 43:861–865, 1980

Wineman NM: Adaptation to multiple sclerosis: the role of social support, functional disability, and perceived uncertainty. Nurs Res 39:294–299, 1990

Zeldow PB, Pavlou M: Physical and psychosocial functioning in multiple sclerosis: descriptions, correlations, and a tentative typology. Br J Med Psychol 61:185–195, 1988

Chapter 7

Disability and Rehabilitation

Carl V. Granger, M.D.,
Margaret M. Hens, M.S., R.N., and
Carol M. Brownscheidle, Ph.D.

Multiple Sclerosis (MS), through demyelination, attacks the integrity of central nervous system (CNS) pathways. As a result, the most common feature of this disease is disability. There are 171,000 people with MS in the United States according to the National Health Interview Survey (1983–1985) (LaPlante 1988). These statistics are based on household interviews of the civilian noninstitutionalized population regarding the prevalence and effects of major health disorders. MS ranks first (40.7%) for individuals needing help in basic life activities, and fourth in causing both limitations in recreational and/or social activities (70.7%) and limitations in major life activities (63.3%).

Unfortunately, there is a tendency to group people disabled by MS into a single category, rather than precisely identify their functional limitations and remaining assets. Because no two MS cases are exactly alike, if we, as a society, are to meet the needs of people with MS better, we have to have sophisticated measures of human function on which to base medical intervention, rehabilitation therapies, and psychological and social support programs.

For the person with disability, attention must be directed to the potential for restoring lost functional abilities through rehabilitation over the long term. There is need to define disability, not by diagnostic labeling, but rather by assessment of functional performance in specific environments. This provides health professionals and policymakers a far better understanding of how to target services to the real needs of the people with disabilities. By focusing on an individual's functional performance (disability and handicap), rather than the organic deficits (impairment), it also becomes possible to capitalize on his or her remaining strengths in a positive manner. Moreover, functional assessment also directs proper attention to the possibilities for modifying the environment in ways that enable functionally impaired people to adapt or to compensate for their limitations.

LONG-TERM CARE ISSUES

In 1990, the National Multiple Sclerosis Society (NMSS) published a position paper entitled, "Long-Term Care Issues in Multiple Sclerosis." They defined long-term care as follows:

> Long-term care is a coordinated continuum of preventive, diagnostic, therapeutic, rehabilitative, supportive and maintenance services that address the health, social, and personal needs of individuals with multiple sclerosis and their families.

NMSS supports the following eight principles in developing and sustaining long-term care of people with MS:

1. Development and implementation of a comprehensive long-term care system are responsibilities that must be shared by governmental and private sector agencies and individuals.
2. Eligibility should be based solely on the need for services.
3. Care settings should be appropriate and the least restrictive.
4. Barrier-free and accessible environments are necessary to assure independence for people with disabilities.
5. The long-term care system should be committed to preserving personal autonomy and maximizing self-determination for all.
6. Providers of care should be appropriately trained and adequately compensated. Family members, friends, neighbors, and volunteers should receive training, respite, counseling, financial incentives, and recognition.
7. A range of rehabilitation services should be available.
8. There should be support for research into the causes and treatment of chronic impairment, the advancement of quality standards for long-term care, and the development of methods for assuring that new findings are incorporated into current practices.

UNIVERSITY AT BUFFALO
MULTIPLE SCLEROSIS SYSTEM

To put these principles into practice, the University at Buffalo Multiple Sclerosis System (UBMSS) was formed in July 1988 as a consortium of facilities and resources with the purpose of providing a long-term, integrated, comprehensive, and caring approach to health and health-related services to individuals with MS and their families. The founding organizations include the William C. Baird MS Research Center of the Millard Fillmore Hospitals, the Bernard B. Hoffman MS Center of The Buffalo General Hospital, and the NMSS Western New York/Northwestern Pennsylvania chapter. Each site has established a cooperative liaison with the State University of New York at Buffalo School of Medicine and Biomedical Sciences—the medical research, education, and training hub of the Western New York community—which forms an umbrella for the triad of service sites.

Successful integration of the patient intake, referral for services, and follow-along processes has been achieved so that the person with MS can access assistance efficiently and minimize the time between their need for services and their delivery. The major mission of the rehabilitation arm of UBMSS is to *address rehabilitation needs and assist people with MS to adapt for optimal functional performance and personal satisfaction with their quality of life.* An important part of this mission is being able to measure disability validly and reliably in order to evaluate the outcomes of the disorder with or without treatment interventions.

Because MS tends to be progressive, the program of care incorporates restorative therapies to recapture lost skills, when this is possible, or uses maintenance strategies to prevent deterioration of current capabilities. All rehabilitation interventions have a common goal: to assess the health and functional states of people with MS in order to strengthen the abilities of the individual and allow living in the community with as high a sense of well-being as possible. The pace of rehabilitation is directed by the realization that any health care program established for a person with MS must be a delicate blending of shifting goals intended to preserve the person's physical abilities and supporting realistic psychosocial adjustment to losses imposed by the neurological disorder. When functional loss is inevitable, the person must be helped to conserve physical and psychosocial abilities at appropriate levels.

During the course of their illness, MS patients may have contacts with primary medical care, neurology, physiatry, urology, nursing, social work, psychiatry and/or psychology, physical therapy, occupational therapy, speech therapy, general medicine, and vocational rehabilitation. Ongoing primary medical care is important because disorders other than those related to MS may crop up, such as hypertension, gastrointestinal disorders, and infections.

GOALS OF REHABILITATION

The goals of rehabilitation are met best through an interdisciplinary team approach that facilitates cross-communication and a dynamic interplay of expertise. It also facilitates continuity and comprehensiveness of care in that over the years the team becomes familiar with the person's needs, thereby providing a greater sense of wholeness. There is also sharing of the gains, the losses, and the memories of life's milestones.

Goal setting in rehabilitation is an ongoing process. Clear and realistic goals developed in collaboration with the person with MS are imperative if gain is to be realized and maintained. Some goals may be precise as in increasing the distance of ambulation with a walker from 10 feet to 50 feet. Other goals may be preventive, as in teaching the patient how to avoid fatigue or contractures or pressure sores that result from immobility.

Every person with MS presents with a different array of problems and time course of events, which makes it impossible to generalize rehabilitation interventions. However, for many people with MS, several problem areas can be expected: fatigue and heat intolerance, need for teaching and counseling about disease phenomena, need to cope with physical and emotional changes induced by the disease, and need to understand and benefit from the use of adaptive equipment.

Fatigue, which is often aggravated by elevation of body temperature or a warm environment, can be a major cause of disability. It is important to realize that, although subjective, fatigue is a symptom that is induced pathophysiologically, not psychologically. It is estimated to occur in more than 80% of people with MS and is characterized as "nerve fiber fatigue" (Reingold 1989). It is to be distinguished from the fatigue that is normally felt as tiredness from overexertion and particularly from fatigue associated with depression (Herndon 1987). Because fatigue is subjective, it cannot be satisfactorily measured. Inability to sustain muscle function may be due to rapid decay in conductivity of demyelinated nerve fibers in the CNS. There is also the possibility of "cognitive tiring," which is associated with the need to consciously and deliberately think through processes to initiate and sustain commonly performed tasks. Many patients relate that they must talk to their feet as if to "tell" them what to do in order to ambulate. Although the Social Security Administration has recognized fatigue as a disabling symptom of MS, it expects physicians to present objective measures for assessing the functional consequences of fatigue.

The debilitating effects of heat are seen with fever, hot bath water, and elevated environmental temperature. For example, a person who can walk 50 feet, feed himself or herself, and dress may be able to walk only 10 feet, lift a utensil for eating for only half a meal, and dress only his or her upper body when exposed to summertime heat. In some cases, the effects of heat intolerance manifest themselves toward late afternoon or evening, when normal body temperature rises a half to a full degree centigrade. Keeping the body cool through the use of air conditioning, energy conservation, and simplification of tasks in daily living is a practical remedy for fatigue and should be a part of any rehabilitative effort.

Ongoing teaching and counseling are necessary for successful management. It should not be assumed that people with MS are knowledgeable about the disease just because they have been given pamphlets to read, attended educational programs, or had the disease for many years. Teaching incorporates skills for managing symptoms and adapting to changes in function, whether it be with adaptive equipment, restorative-maintenance therapies, or assistance of another person. Although teaching and counseling are integral to the rehabilitation program, it must always be remembered that the patients' abilities to integrate new information and call on their repertoire of daily living skills may be diminished by stress. Stress may be in the form of anxiety, depression, fatigue, or even cognitive activity. It is not uncommon to note reduced abilities in short-term memory, insight, judgment, and problem-solving skills. Enrollment in peer groups has helped many people with MS learn to cope with stress.

Adaptive equipment has become more available in response to advances in technology as well as increased numbers of people with impairments and disabilities. There are many variations of environmental control devices that may be activated with the slightest physical movement or even from a person's breath. Communication aids connected to computers have opened up opportunities for verbal interaction by severely limited individuals. Consequently, options for vocational and leisure time participation have expanded.

Equipment for mobility, such as wheelchairs, canes, walkers, crutches, and orthoses (braces) should be prescribed by a physician who is knowledgeable about the ways that these devices may enhance a person's life-style. For example, although not needed at all times, a wheelchair may be recommended and prescribed when the person needs to travel over distances that might cause fatigue. A wheelchair may be recommended for the person going to an event in order that by conserving energy he or she may derive more enjoyment. A person with MS should always be measured for adaptive equipment. Ill-fitting mobility aids can lead to improper seating position and further fatigue and postural strain on the spine.

There are literally hundreds of different aids to daily living. Long-handled sponges, special utensils, writing aids, slide-out cabinets, and extra-long shoehorns are examples of devices that help disabled people care for themselves and circumvent environmental obstacles more easily. Bathroom equipment such as raised toilet seats, shower benches, hand-held shower heads, and tub lifts are additional examples of aids designed for making bathing and toileting easier. There are many catalogs and retail outlets that carry adaptive clothing. Velcro closures, false backs, and wrap-around garments have been demanded from the clothing industry and the response has been positive, stylish, and attentive to the appeal of different age groups. Adaptive equipment not only increases independence but satisfies one's sense of well-being. How frustrating it is to try to button a shirt for a half an hour when a buttonhook can be used one-handed and rather quickly!

Rehabilitation treatments for specific MS symptoms are beyond the scope of this chapter and are well documented elsewhere (Ahearn and Schwetz 1985; Cobble et al. 1988; Conomy et al. 1986; Erickson et al. 1989; Kraft et al. 1986). Management of the symptoms of MS may diminish their adverse impact on functional capabilities and thereby prevent unnecessary disability. For example, it may not be necessary to overmedicate the person with mild-to-moderate spasticity if that symptom is only an annoyance. In fact, some spasticity may permit the patient to perform a standing pivot when transferring out of a chair. However, lower-limb spasticity should not go unattended to the point at which amputation is the only solution left because of severe contractures, which may be associated with pressure sores of the skin and problems of maintaining perineal hygiene. Bowel and bladder dysfunction may have profound effects on MS patients' life-styles. People with MS may abuse laxatives and be in a state of alternating constipation and diarrhea; patients with diarrhea may be manifesting intolerance to lactose in their diet. Problems of bladder control may be interrelated with difficulty in mobility, such that patients may confine themselves in order to stay close to toilet facilities. Patients placed on diuretics for control of hypertension may find that bladder incontinence has become an unmanageable problem.

FUNCTIONAL ASSESSMENT MEASURES

Accurate measures of a person's levels of independence in the performance of personal care activities of daily living and mobility (e.g., eating, grooming, bathing, dressing, toileting, managing bladder and bowel continence, and locomotion), instrumental activities of daily living (e.g., telephoning, taking medications, shopping, doing laundry, cooking, and obtaining transportation), and cognitive-social tasks of daily living (e.g., problem solving, communication, memory, decision making, establishing and maintaining relationships, and emotional adaptability) are crucial to the patient, rehabilitation program, health care system, and society at large. Documentation of objective, quantified performance in activities of daily living provides a distinct picture of what the patient can do and what someone else must do for him or her (i.e., burden of care or need for assistance). To say to a patients "You seem better" is not the same as saying "You now provide 50% of the effort of dressing yourself as compared to 25% 1 month ago." Reality keeps unrealistic perceptions at bay. Documented functional data are imperative for disability claims and benefits. Accurate measurement of functional performance also impacts greatly on the need for institutionalization and the assistance required of caregivers.

Functional assessment is a method for describing abilities and limitations in order to measure an individual's use of the various skills included in performing tasks necessary to daily living, leisure activities, vocational pursuits, social interactions, and other required behaviors. A profile developed from functional assessment data provides the clinician with a framework for orderly review of needs at the individual and societal levels. It is possible to compare changes in status over periods of time by assessing function at appropriate intervals to determine whether social roles have been influenced by professional interventions of health care, rehabilitation, education, or psychological and social counseling. The measures can describe changes both for individuals and for groups of individuals (Granger 1990).

At the national level, the need for a more unified and rigorous approach to functional assessment has been identified. The 1982 annual report of the National Council for the Handicapped called for common terminology, a unifying conceptual framework, more field research, and greater communication among investigators (Joe 1984). Internationally, similar needs and priorities are recognized. The United Nations Inquiry Regarding Assessment of Disability Legislation pinpointed a worldwide need for more research to document the nature and frequency of disability and to provide the means for documenting human needs and service program effectiveness (United Nations Department of International Economics and Social Affairs 1986). The *International Classification of Impairments, Disabilities, and Handicaps* (ICIDH) (called "the Disablement Model") was published by the World Health

Organization (1980). It sparked a surge of conceptual and taxonomic progress in functional assessment research. In 1984, Granger and Gresham edited the volume, *Functional Assessment in Rehabilitation Medicine,* which presented the state-of-the-art and technical information needed for a revolutionary shift in attitudes regarding disability and disabled people (Joe 1984).

According to ICIDH, *disability* is

> Any restriction or lack of ability to perform an activity in the manner or within the range considered normal for a human being. Disability is concerned with abilities, in the form of composite activities and behaviors, that are generally accepted as essential components of everyday life. Examples include disturbances in behaving in an appropriate manner, in personal care (such as excretory control and the ability to wash and feed oneself), in the performance of other activities of daily living, and in locomotor activities (such as the ability to walk). (Duckworth 1984, p. 10)

Handicap is

> A disadvantage for a given individual that limits or prevents the fulfillment of a role that is normal (depending upon age, sex, and social and cultural factors) for that individual. Handicap is concerned with the value attached to an individual's situation or experience when it departs from the norm. It is characterized by a discordance between the individual's performance or status and the expectations of the individual himself or of the particular group of which he is a member. Handicap thus represents socialization of an impairment or disability and, as such, it reflects the consequences for the individual—cultural, economic, and environmental—that stem from the presence of impairment and disability. Disadvantage arises from failure or inability to conform to the expectations or norms of the individual's universe. Handicap thus occurs when there is interference with the ability to sustain what might be designated as "survival roles." (Duckworth 1984, p. 10)

Bergner (1989) examined health status measures used in clinical research. In response to naive clinical investigators who desire a single best measure, she pointed out the bitter truth that there is no gold standard, nor is there ever likely to be one; and it

may not be desirable to have one. Measurement of disability—
restriction or lack in performance of usual and expected activities—is an important domain of health status measurement.
Even in clinical trials, use of multidimensional health status measures in noncurable disorders could detect intended beneficial
and even unintended adverse effects of treatment. Although clinical trials are intended to examine a medical outcome, in the case
of MS change in neurological status, it must be realized that
therapy may affect aspects of a person's life that are not strictly
medical. To date, efforts toward formalized functional assessment methodology in rehabilitation medicine have produced a
number of specific "instruments" that can be grouped into three
basic types:

1. The *global instruments* provide an overall functional profile of
   a patient that is relatively comprehensive with variable levels
   of detail regarding component items. Examples of global instruments include PULSES (Moskowitz and McCann 1957)
   the Functional Life Scale (FLS; Sarno et al. 1973), and the
   Functional Status Index (FSI; Jette 1980).
2. The scales most frequently used are the *activities of daily living
   (ADL) scales*, which emphasize achievement of independence
   in self-care and mobility. Prototypes of these scales include
   the Katz Index of ADL (Katz et al. 1963), the Barthel Index (BI;
   Mahoney and Barthel 1965), the Kenny Self-Care Evaluation
   (Gresham et al. 1980b), and the Functional Independence
   Measure (FIM; Granger and Hamilton 1992).
3. There are a number of *categorical instruments* designed to address the unique functional profiles of patients with a particular disease or condition, such as the Quadriplegia Index of
   Function (QIF; Gresham et al. 1980a) and the Minimum Record of Disability for Multiple Sclerosis (MRD) (International
   Federation of Multiple Sclerosis Societies 1985).

Table 7–1 illustrates the relationship between the functional
assessment approach and development of treatment strategies
for a person with chronic MS. Repeated evaluations of functional
status over time make treatment more effective and efficient by
addressing problems that the patient views as most limiting

Table 7-1. Terminology, clinical manifestations, and treatment of multiple sclerosis, using the ICIDH model of chronic disease

Terminology	Expression	Clinical manifestations	Treatment
Pathology CNS plaques	Demyelination	CSF analysis; CNS imaging; evoked potential testing	Immunosuppression; anti-inflammatory
Impairment and/or functional limitations	Signs and symptoms	Weakness; spasticity; ataxia; sensory loss; fatigability; heat intolerance; neurogenic bladder or bowel; visual deficits; pressure sores; etc.	Graded rest and activity; antispasmodics; physical therapy; occupational therapy; braces or splints; nerve blocks; catheter or suppository
Disability	Inability to perform tasks	Reduced walking; incontinence; reduced self-care; reduced seeing	As above, plus wheelchair; adaptive devices; environmental adjustments; counseling
Handicap	Reduction in expected social role performance	Job loss; changed sexual attitude and/or function; changed spousal role	As above, plus social work; community resources

Note. ICIDH = International Classification of Impairments, Disabilities, and Handicaps (World Health Organization 1980)

(Granger 1984). Thus the health care provider can improve compliance and thereby enhance the patient's quality of life.

For patients with MS, functional assessment is a logical approach to determining need for services (Granger 1981). Disability imposes burdens of physical care and psychological distress on the individual and the caregivers. Analysis of the relationships between instruments or scales currently used to assess disability and their ability to predict the burdens of physical care and psychological distress is imperative. This is especially true if such scales are to be used for evaluating treatment options or for allocating long-term rehabilitative and supportive services that are intended to relieve these burdens by promoting independent functioning of the individual and appropriate use of environmental supports.

Assessment instruments used to measure disability, handicap, and psychological symptoms should provide precise information regarding important clinical changes in patients. They have been used in many clinical investigations involving subjects with MS and a variety of other chronic health conditions (e.g., stroke, spinal cord and head injury, arthritis, and amputation). Usually they are used independently, but on occasion with one or two other measures (Gresham et al. 1980b; Jacelon 1986). Seven functional assessment instruments used to assess MS patients are summarized in Table 7–2 and discussed below.

- *Expanded Disability Status Scale:* For nearly 30 years neurologists have been using the neurological Functional Systems (FS) and Disability Status Scales of Kurtzke (DSS) (Kurtzke 1961). DSS scores are derived from FS descriptors of CNS dysfunction. Steps 1 through 6 are used for ambulatory people and steps 7 through 10 for nonambulatory people. The Kurtzke system reflects neurological impairment status from which disability is inferred rather than measured. The Kurtzke scales, including the expanded version of DSS (EDSS; Kurtzke 1983), are included in the MRD.
- *Barthel Index:* Until recently, the Barthel Index (BI) was probably the best known functional assessment instrument in medical rehabilitation settings in the United States. It was

Table 7–2. Summary of seven functional assessment instruments

Instrument	Developer	Uses	Scale range
Expanded Disability Status Scale (EDSS)	Kurtzke (1983)	Classify the effects of neurological dysfunction, particularly on ambulation	Best = 0 Worst = 10 10 levels
Barthel Index	Mahoney and Barthel (1965)	Classify and follow patient progress during rehabilitation	Best = 100 Worst = 0 3–4 levels
Functional Independence Measure (FIM)	National Rehabilitation Task Force (Hamilton et al. 1987)	Classify disability of individuals for outcome measurement	Best = 126 Worst = 18 7 levels
Incapacity Status Scale (ISS)	Kurtzke and Granger (1980)	Classify disability of people with multiple sclerosis (MS) for clinical and research purposes	Best = 0 Worst = 64 5 levels
Environmental Status Scale (ESS)	International group (Mellerup et al. 1981)	Classify social dysfunction of people with MS for clinical and research purposes	Best = 0 Worst = 35 5 levels
Brief Symptom Inventory (BSI)	Derogatis (1977)	Characterize psychological distress	9 subscores 3 summary scores
Sickness Impact Profile (SIP)	Bergner et al. (1981)	Characterize change in health status in 12 domains	12 domains 2 globals Best = 0% Worst = 100%

developed by Mahoney and Barthel in 1965. The original instrument contained 10 items and was scored in intervals of 5 points to a maximum score of 100. The preferential weighting assigned by the BI to continence and mobility represents a professionally shrewd prioritization of the most crucial activities of daily living skills. The BI has been found to be simple to use and has well-established reliability, validity, and precision (Gresham et al. 1980b). One limitation of the index, however, is that the intervals between points are not equal, thus a change in the number of points received by two different clients does not necessarily reflect an equal change in disability. Further, communication and mental status deficits are not identified in the scale. Granger et al. (1979) developed a four-level, slightly expanded adaptation of the BI and incorporated it into the Long-Range Evaluation System (LRES; Granger and McNamara 1984).

- *Functional Independence Measure:* The Functional Independence Measure (FIM; Granger and Hamilton 1992; Hamilton et al. 1987) is a part of the Uniform Data System for Medical Rehabilitation (UDSMR) (Granger et al. 1986, 1990; Hamilton et al. 1987; Keith et al. 1987). FIM is a part of the data set produced by a National Rehabilitation Task Force originated by the American Congress of Rehabilitation Medicine and the American Academy of Physical Medicine and Rehabilitation in 1983. UDSMR contains a minimum data set composed of demographic, diagnostic, functional, and cost information. The key component is the FIM, which incorporated items of the BI, but is more sensitive and inclusive. Data collected by the FIM is consistent in terminology and is used by clinicians and researchers to track patients from the initiation of a treatment intervention through discharge and follow-up. The FIM has been tested extensively in multiple rehabilitation facilities and has been found to be satisfactory in reliability, validity, feasibility, and precision.

- *Incapacity Status Scale:* The Incapacity Status Scale (ISS) was constructed by Kurtzke and Granger to assess disability. It was developed as a part of the MRD under the impetus of the International Federation of Multiple Sclerosis Societies (1985).

The purpose was to promote a minimum record system, establish uniformity of data collection, and provide standardized profiles of the main dysfunctions associated with MS for comparing clinical and research results (International Federation of Multiple Sclerosis Societies 1985; Slater and Raun 1984).

- *Environmental Status Scale:* The Environmental Status Scale (ESS) was developed by Mellerup et al. (1981) to assess handicap. The ESS measures seven areas of social performance or need: work status, financial/economic status, personal residence/home, personal assistance, transportation, community assistance, and social activity. The 1985 version of the MRD (International Federations of Multiple Sclerosis Societies 1985) contains the ISS and ESS. This composite scale is the result of refinements and statistical testing by LaRocca et al. (1984).

- *Brief Symptom Inventory:* Another important dimension of health status is one's perception of well-being. Subjective and emotional symptomatology are important to assess even though they may be less likely to be influenced directly by treatment. Also, they may improve or worsen in directions that are not necessarily the same as those indicated by measurements of physical functioning. The Brief Symptom Inventory (BSI; Derogatis and Melisaratos 1983) is a measure of psychological symptomatology in which influences of physical infirmity are not overly weighted. It is a 53-item version of the Symptom Checklist—90 (SCL-90; Derogatis et al. 1974), a well-established self-report instrument for assessing psychiatric symptoms among inpatients or outpatients. The BSI uses a multiple choice format for responding to inquiries about cognitive, behavioral, affective, and physiological difficulties. Standardization and psychometric data concerning validation of subscales are provided in an accompanying manual (Derogatis 1977). The BSI is easily administered and scored to assess the extent of psychological distress.

- *Sickness Impact Profile:* A different approach to measurement of health status is offered by the Sickness Impact Profile (SIP; Bergner et al. 1981). The SIP is a performance-oriented functional status measure that provides a profile of functional problems using respondent self-report. The SIP has 136 items that assess a broad range of ADLs within 12 functional areas. The instrument has a demonstrated sensitivity both to change in functional status that occurs over time within an illness group and to differences in functional status between illness groups. The reliability and high levels of both test-retest reliability and internal consistency have been demonstrated. Scores on the SIP range from 0 to 100, with higher scores representing greater disability. In an unreported study (Minden S, unpublished observations, March 1989) of 50 patients (62% female; average age 40 years), there was an overall score of 25 for patients with an average DSS score of 4.2 (0 being the best; 10 the worst). The higher level of functional limitations among these patients tended to occur in the domains of work, recreation and pastimes, home management, ambulation, and alertness. The SIP is particularly useful for the MS population in the mild to moderate rather than severe disability categories.

FUNCTIONAL ASSESSMENT STUDIES

Although there has been progress in developing a conceptual framework for measuring disability as a subset of health status, further work is needed to establish the validity of related scales in predicting the burden of physical care and/or the subjective perception of well-being. One direct measure of the burden of physical care is the amount of time that others spend assisting the disabled person with daily living tasks. Needs of a home care population can be studied in terms of the number of tasks in which help was given and comparable BI scores (Fortinsky et al. 1981).

A recent study (Granger et al. 1990) of the predictive validity of functional assessment analyzed assessment instruments in combination with demographic data to determine which may provide a realistic basis for establishing the burden of care relative to MS. The study included scales for limb functioning, satisfaction with life in general, the BI, the ISS, the FIM, the ESS, and the BSI. A "help at home journal" was developed that listed the personal care activities typically expected to require assistance from another person, whether family, friend, or personal care aide. These activities included feeding, bathing, dressing, bladder and bowel management, and mobility tasks. The conclusions from this study were that the ISS and the BI distinguish crudely between degrees of assistance, whereas the FIM is more precise. Except for the item that measures visual ability, ISS items were redundant to those in the FIM or did not contribute uniquely to prediction of the number of minutes of help that the subjects required. Therefore, FIM is strengthened by addition of the ISS visual item plus a measure of the sensorimotor functions of the upper limbs. There was a strong relationship between the FIM and the amount of care that the patients received at home. With the BSI and the ESS, the FIM contributed to predicting the patient's level of satisfaction with life in general.

WHICH FUNCTIONS SHOULD BE ASSESSED?

Clinicians must access and integrate information regarding disability and handicap to understand the myriad effects of MS on activities and behaviors that are components of everyday living (e.g., bowel and bladder function, personal grooming, and locomotor activities) and on the ability of the person to meet social role expectations.

Ware (1987) has identified five generic health concepts: physical functioning, mental functioning, social functioning, role functioning, and perception of well-being (Table 7–3). These multidimensions of functioning and well-being must be recognized in the measurement of health. *Physical functioning* is commonly measured in terms of performance of personal care activities and

Table 7–3. Comprehensive outcome measures for multiple sclerosis according to domains of health status measurement

Physical functioning	Includes performance of simple self-care to more physically demanding activities
Mental functioning	Includes cognitive and affective functioning
Social functioning	Includes interactions with other persons
Role functioning	Includes societal roles and functions
Perception of well-being	Subjective feelings

Source. Adapted from Ware 1987.

more strenuous physical activities. *Mental functioning* encompasses feelings that may or may not be revealed in behaviors; therefore, these measures include both behavioral dysfunction and subjective symptoms of psychological distress. *Social functioning* encompasses person-to-person contacts and social support networks. *Role functioning* refers to the capacity to perform usual role activities of employment, schoolwork, and/or household responsibilities. *Perception of well-being* is derived from self-ratings based on the person's subjective notions.

UBMSS has developed protocols for collecting data related to health and functional status according to Ware's domains of health status measurement. The demographic and functional assessment items below provide a profile for each person with MS:

1. Marital, employment, living situation statuses
2. Financial and health insurance information
3. Functional status—how independently ADLs are performed
4. Social activity, participation in leisure and recreational endeavors, and trips outside the home

This information from functional assessment is important for clinical management to

1. Monitor a patient's progress (or lack thereof) over time
2. Measure the effects of specific treatment regimens
3. Propose alternative methods of therapy
4. Coordinate community resources and services with patient needs
5. Make placement decisions
6. Assess rehabilitation outcomes in relation to costs to the patient, as well as to the health care system

CASE EXAMPLE

The following case example illustrates how data collected as part of a patient's continuous medical record may be used as a basis for deciding clinical management issues and implementing support services.

S.B. is a 49-year-old woman who experienced right lower-limb paralysis and numbness in 1973. She was asymptomatic until optic neuritis caused temporary blindness in 1983. This was followed by a short period of intention tremor of the upper limbs. In 1988 she awoke barely able to speak. She was treated with a 10-day course of steroids, which led to improvement, but dysarthria persisted and worsened with fatigue. For the next 2 years her only medication was amantadine, for fatigue.

S.B. has been followed in UBMSS since 1988. Between annual formal assessments, the coordinator has maintained telephone contact with her. Table 7–4 illustrates highlights from her functional assessments, 2 years apart. This assessment profile is the basis for developing a plan of care that includes physical, mental, social, and role functioning, plus the subjective sense of well-being. From the assessment in 1988, it is apparent that S.B. was independent in personal care and mobility, visually limited, and not participating in a rehabilitation program. Her level of psychological distress was high, and she was separated from her husband. She was a full-time student in a business school, and her social contacts were limited. She expressed that she was "more satisfied than not with life in general."

The more recent assessment (1990) documents that S.B. remained independent in personal care and mobility. She had attended 24 speech therapy sessions in the previous year. Divorce proceedings had been completed, and her level of psychological distress had lessened to a normal range. She had completed her business degree and was employable, but unable to find work. Her social contacts had increased. She was managing on public assistance. She expressed that she was "not satisfied with life in general."

Comparison of the assessments over a 2-year span indicates that S.B. gained 1 point in the FIM motor score. This gain was attributable to being able to go up and down stairs without a handrail. In particular she had been limited by fatigue, which had been improved with prescription of amantadine. Fatigue also aggravated her dysarthria. She was referred for speech therapy and counseling with a social worker. Additionally, the nurse coordinator provided education about features of MS and energy conservation techniques. After ophthalmologic consultation, her visual acuity improved, but the dysarthria slightly worsened,

Table 7–4. Highlights of functional assessment for patient S.B., 2 years apart

Assessment	1988	1990
Physical functioning		
Number of outpatient treatment visits	0	24
Vision	Unable to read newsprint	With corrective lenses, able to read newsprint
FIM motor score	90/91	91/91
Mental functioning		
FIM cognitive score	35/35	34/35
BSI total score	198/150	145/150
Social functioning		
Marital status	Separated	Divorced
Living arrangement	Recently moved, parents and son	Parents and son
Social visits at home, past month	3	6
Social trips outside home, past month	9	30
Role functioning		
Employment status	Student	Business school graduate, unemployed
Financial status	No MS-related financial problem	Receiving public assistance
Transportation access	Drives automobile	Drives automobile
Sense of well-being		
Satisfaction with life in general	More satisfied than not satisfied	Not satisfied

Note. FIM = Functional Independence Measure (Hamilton et al. 1987); BSI = Brief Symptom Inventory (Derogatis and Melisaratos 1983); MS = multiple sclerosis

Outpatient treatment visits are counted over the past year.

FIM motor score is based on 13 items of self-care, mobility, sphincter control, and locomotion scored from dependence to independence (1–7).

FIM cognitive score is based on 5 items of communication and social cognition scored from dependence to independence (1–7).

BSI total score is based on summing three subscores of general severity index, positive symptom distress index, and positive symptom total. Normal scores for each of the three is 50, with 60 representing one standard deviation.

Satisfaction with life in general may be answered as "very satisfied," "fairly well satisfied," "more satisfied than not satisfied," or "not satisfied."

accounting for the 1-point drop in the FIM cognitive score. S.B. increased her social contacts both in her own home and outside. She became divorced and maintained living arrangements with her parents and her son.

Regarding role functioning, S.B. was graduated from business school with honors, but was unable to find a job despite assistance from the social worker and the vocational rehabilitation counselor. Her financial situation changed because of her divorce and unemployment. Her subjective sense of well-being declined to "not being satisfied with life in general."

Analysis of the assessment results enabled the rehabilitation team members to appreciate the dynamic interplay between life changes and planned interventions. It might have been expected that as her psychological distress lessened, S.B.'s sense of well-being would have increased, particularly as her physical functioning was maintained. However, S.B. was not content with living with her parents, she remained frustrated with unemployment despite a straight-A average in school, and she did not have the financial resources to make alternative living arrangements. She believed that her dysarthria was the main reason she was unable to secure a job. Thus she was feeling and functioning better physically and developed a coping mechanism for psychological distress, but remained frustrated in not reaching her goals in role functioning. Her plans included seeking opportunities for volunteerism in order to increase her contacts with the business community.

SUMMARY

People with MS, as well as their families and caregivers, may benefit from a center that combines a neurological and rehabilitation orientation because

1. Many symptoms associated with the disease are chronic and are not amenable to short-term management.
2. The unpredictable nature of MS requires individualized periodic health and functional monitoring so that problems are promptly identified and treatments instituted and evaluated.
3. Ongoing monitoring of care is vital to prevent complications

(e.g., pressure sores, excessive muscle spasticity, deep venous thrombosis, and urological and bowel dysfunction) and increased disability, which increase dependency and costs of care.
4. Accenting maintenance of function and, when necessary, adaptation to a change in function focuses on ability rather than disability and fosters patient participation in long-term health management.
5. The nature of the data collected about center patients will improve clinicians' insights into common problems and circumstances of people with MS.
6. Data about patients are the bases for analyzing service needs and the relationships between costs and benefits in the comprehensive management of people with MS.
7. A central organization for coordinating care facilitates comprehensive and efficient care of patients who have complex and interacting problems.

REFERENCES

Ahearn JP, Schwetz KM: Comprehensive supportive therapy in multiple sclerosis. Semin Neurol 5:146–154, 1985

Bergner M: Quality of life, health status, and clinical research. Med Care 27:S148–S156, 1989

Bergner M, Bobbitt RA, Carter WB, et al: The sickness impact profile: development and final revision of a health status measure. Med Care 19:787–805, 1981

Cobble ND, Wangaard C, Kraft GH, et al: Rehabilitation of the patient with multiple sclerosis, in Rehabilitation Medicine Principles and Practice. Edited by DeLisa J. Philadelphia, JB Lippincott, 1988, pp 612–634

Conomy JP, Bhasin C, Fischer J, et al: The experience of the Mellen Center for Multiple Sclerosis Treatment and Research at the Cleveland Clinic Foundation. Paper presented at the Multiple Sclerosis Symposium, Scientific Advances and Interdisciplinary Care, at The Cleveland Clinic Educational Foundation, Cleveland, OH, March, 1986

Derogatis LR: The SCL-90 Manual I: Scoring, Administration and Procedure for the SCL-90. Baltimore, MD, Clinical Psychometric Research, 1977

Derogatis LR, Melisaratos N: The Brief Symptom Inventory: an introductory report. Psychol Med 13:595–605, 1983

Derogatis LR, Lipman RS, Rickels K, et al: The Hopkins Symptom Checklist (HSCL): a self-report symptom inventory. Behav Sci 19:1–15, 1974

Duckworth D: The need for a standard terminology and classification of disablement, in Functional Assessment in Rehabilitation Medicine. Edited by Granger CV, Gresham GE. Baltimore, MD, Williams & Wilkins, 1984, p 10

Erickson RP, Lie MR, Wineinger MA: Rehabilitation in multiple sclerosis. Mayo Clin Proc 64:818–828, 1989

Fortinsky RH, Granger CV, Seltzer GB: The use of functional assessment in understanding home care needs. Med Care 19:489–497, 1981

Granger CV: Assessment of functional status: a model for multiple sclerosis. Acta Neurol Scand 64 (suppl 87):40–47, 1981

Granger CV: A conceptual model for functional assessment, in Functional Assessment in Rehabilitation Medicine. Edited by Granger CV, Gresham GE. Baltimore, MD, Williams & Wilkins, 1984, pp 14–26

Granger CV: Health accounting: functional assessment of the long-term patient, in Krusen's Handbook of Physical Medicine and Rehabilitation, 4th Edition. Edited by Kottke FJ, Lehmann JF. Philadelphia, PA, WB Saunders, 1990, pp 270–282

Granger CV, Gresham GE: Preface, in Functional Assessment in Rehabilitation Medicine. Edited by Granger CV, Gresham GE. Baltimore, MD, Williams & Wilkins, 1984, pp ix–x

Granger CV, Hamilton BB: UDS report: the uniform data system for medical rehabilitation report for first admissions for 1990. Am J Phys Med Rehabil 71:108–113, 1992

Granger CV, McNamara MA: Functional assessment utilization: the Long-Range Evaluation System (LRES), in Functional Assessment in Rehabilitation Medicine. Edited by Granger CV, Gresham GE. Baltimore, MD, Williams & Wilkins, 1984, pp 99–121

Granger CV, Albrecht GL, Hamilton BB: Outcome of comprehensive medical rehabilitation: measurement of PULSES Profile and the Barthel Index. Arch Phys Med Rehabil 60:145–154, 1979

Granger CV, Hamilton BB, Keith RA, et al: Advances in functional assessment for medical rehabilitation, in Topics in Geriatric Rehabilitation, Vol. 1. Edited by Lewis CB. Rockville, MD, Aspen Publishing, 1986, pp 59–74

Granger CV, Cotter AC, Hamilton BB, et al: Functional assessment scales: study of persons with multiple sclerosis. Arch Phys Med Rehabil 71:870–875, 1990

Gresham GE, Labi ML, Dittmar SS, et al: Quadriplegia Index of Function (abstract). Arch Phys Med Rehabil 61:493, 1980a

Gresham GE, Phillips TF, Labi ML: ADL status in stroke: relative merits of three standard indexes. Arch Phys Med Rehabil 61:355–358, 1980b

Hamilton BB, Granger CV, Sherwin FS, et al: A uniform national data system for medical rehabilitation, in Rehabilitation Outcomes: Analysis and Measurement. Edited by Fuhrer MJ. Baltimore, MD, Paul H. Brookes, 1987, pp 137–147

Herndon RM: Fatigue in MS. Paper presented at the Symposium on Multiple Sclerosis, Buffalo, NY, May 1987

International Federation of Multiple Sclerosis Societies: MRD: Minimal Record of Disability for Multiple Sclerosis. New York, National Multiple Sclerosis Society, 1985

Jacelon CS: The Barthel Index and other indices of functional ability. Rehabilitation Nursing 11:9–11, 1986

Jette AM: Functional Status Index: reliability of a chronic disease evaluation instrument. Arch Phys Med Rehabil 61:395–401, 1980

Joe T: Foreword, in Functional Assessment in Rehabilitation Medicine. Edited by Granger CV, Gresham GE. Baltimore, MD, Williams & Wilkins, 1984, pp vii–viii

Katz S, Ford AB, Moskowitz RW, et al: Studies of illness in the aged: the index of ADL: A standardized measure of biological and psychosocial function. JAMA 185:914–919, 1963

Keith RA, Granger CV, Hamilton BB, et al: The Functional Independence Measure: a new tool for rehabilitation, in Advances in Clinical Rehabilitation, Vol 1. Edited by Eisenberg MG, Grzesiak RC. New York, Springer, 1987, pp 6–18

Kraft GH, Freal JC, Coryell JK: Disability, disease duration, and rehabilitation service needs in multiple sclerosis: patient perspectives. Arch Phys Med Rehabil 67:164–168, 1986

Kurtzke JF: On the evaluation of disability in multiple sclerosis. Neurology 11:686–694, 1961

Kurtzke JF: Rating neurological impairment in multiple sclerosis: an expanded disability status scale (EDSS). Neurology 33:1444–1452, 1983

LaPlante MP: Data on Disability From the National Health Interview Survey, 1983–85: In InfoUse Report. Washington DC, U.S. National Institute on Disability and Rehabilitation Research, 1988

LaRocca MG, Scheinbrg LC, Slater RJ, et al: Field testing of a minimal record of disability in multiple sclerosis: the United States and Canada. Acta Neurol Scand Suppl 101:126–138, 1984

Mahoney FI, Barthel DW: Functional evaluation: the Barthel Index. Maryland State Medical Journal 14:61–65, 1965

Mellerup E, Fog T, Niels R, et al: The socioeconomic scale. Acta Neurol Scand 64 (suppl 87):130–138, 1981

Moskowitz E, McCann CB: Classification of disability in the chronically ill and aging. Journal of Chronic Disease 5:342–346, 1957

National Multiple Sclerosis Society: Long-Term Care Issues in Multiple Sclerosis: A Position Paper. New York, National Multiple Sclerosis Society, 1990

Reingold SC: Fatigue and multiple sclerosis. MS Quarterly Report 8(3):34–36, 1989

Sarno JE, Sarno MT, Levita E: The Functional Life Scale. Arch Phys Med Rehabil 54:214–220, 1973

Slater RJ, Raun NE (eds): Symposium on a Minimum Record of Disability for Multiple Sclerosis. Copenhagen, Munksgaard. International Federation of Multiple Sclerosis Societies, 1984

United Nations Department of International Economics and Social Affairs: Disability: Situation, Strategies and Policies. New York, UN Agent, 1986

Ware JE: Standards for validating health measures: definition and content. Journal of Chronic Disease 40:473–480, 1987

World Health Organization: International Classification of Impairments, Disabilities, and Handicaps. Geneva, Switzerland, World Health Organization, 1980

Chapter 8

Patients' Advocacy Groups and Support Associations in Multiple Sclerosis: The National Multiple Sclerosis Society

Stephen C. Reingold, Ph.D.

The National Multiple Sclerosis Society (NMSS) is the only voluntary health agency in the United States that provides a nationwide program of services, advocacy, and research for the country's estimated 350,000 people with multiple sclerosis (MS). From its beginnings in 1946, NMSS has expanded greatly. In 1991 alone, NMSS raised more than $75 million to fund its services and programs relating to MS, which, after epilepsy, is the most prevalent neurological disorder among young adults in North America.

ORIGINS AND FOUNDING

NMSS was founded almost single-handedly by Sylvia Lawry, who, in an attempt to find help for her brother who had been diagnosed with MS, placed a classified ad in the *New York Times* in 1945:

> Multiple sclerosis. Will anyone recovered from it please communicate with patient. T272 Times.

Ms. Lawry received an overwhelming response, not from anyone who had recovered from MS, but from individuals with the disease, their families, and friends, who were also seeking help. As a result, in the spring of 1946 a group of the first respondents to the ad formed the Association for the Advancement of Research on Multiple Sclerosis (AARMS) and began cooperatively to raise money for research and services for people with MS.

In 1947, a group of lay and medical and scientific volunteers held their first joint meeting. At this meeting, they changed the organization's name to the National Multiple Sclerosis Society, funded the first research grant (to Dr. Elvin Kabat at Columbia University, for studies on immunological factors of MS, in the amount of $64,350), and chartered the first local chapters of the organization in Western Connecticut and Southern California.

Over the years the organization has grown enormously. Today (1992), there are 140 chapters and branches in the United States, serving virtually every community in the country, and NMSS funds more than $10,600,000 in research and research training programs. NMSS has a current membership of nearly 400,000, including over 170,000 individuals with MS.

NMSS has had significant influence on research and public policy related to MS, neurological disorders, and chronic disabilities more generally, in the United States and abroad. Among the more important roles it has played is key leadership in encouraging federal legislation, which, in 1950, established the National Institute of Neurological and Communicative Disorders and Stroke (now the National Institute of Neurological Disorders and Stroke) within the National Institutes of Health (NIH). NMSS has also been instrumental in founding national multiple sclerosis societies in 33 countries around the world. These organizations, serving more than 2 million people with MS worldwide, were brought together in 1967 under the International Federation of Multiple Sclerosis Societies, an umbrella organization located in London.

MISSION AND GOALS

Since its inception, NMSS has been dedicated to the prevention, treatment, and eventual cure of multiple sclerosis and to improving the quality of life for people with MS and their families. To accomplish these goals, NMSS works to

- Stimulate, coordinate, and support research into the cause, prevention, diagnosis, treatment, and cure of the disease

- Seek out and disseminate reliable information and medical and scientific opinion concerning MS and its treatment and communicate this in formation to people with MS, the medical and scientific community, and the general public
- Provide direct services to MS patients and their families
- Develop and promote public policy to help individuals affected by MS

To accomplish these goals, NMSS conducts vigorous fundraising, marketing, and public relations campaigns at national and local levels to raise necessary funds and heighten public awareness of the disease.

RESEARCH PROGRAMS

With the recognition that insight into MS and a cure can come only through basic and applied research, NMSS has, since its inception, supported a wide-ranging program of biomedical research related to the disease.

Research at NMSS is characterized by a high-quality peer review system that evaluates research proposals on scientific merit and on relevance to questions about MS. Research administration is coordinated centrally at the national headquarters in New York City, and grants are distributed without regional considerations: only the best programs are funded at research and medical institutions around the country and abroad. Funding decisions are closely coordinated with NIH—the only other agency that provides significant MS research support—to prevent dual funding of overlapping projects.

As the funds available have increased over the years, NMSS has been able to support an increasing spectrum of research and training programs. Currently, dollars may be allocated for

- *Basic or fundamental research,* often on animal models of MS.
- *Clinical or applied research* involving people with MS, which ranges in scope from primary questions about basic biological function to clinical trials to examine the safety and efficacy of new therapeutic agents.

- *Patient management and rehabilitation grants,* which provide support for projects aimed at symptomatic problems of MS (e.g., spasticity, fatigue, and cognitive and affective disorders related to MS) and testing of new strategies aimed at improving the quality of life of those with MS.
- *Pilot research grants,* supporting small, short-term projects to allow an investigator to collect preliminary data on novel hypotheses, which would allow preparation of a full grant application at a later date.
- *Health services research projects,* designed to allow collection of data relevant to service delivery, demographics, and quality of care for people with MS. Data from this program provide background needed to help effect change in entitlement programs, insurance coverage, and legislation related to MS and disabilities in general.
- *Postdoctoral fellowships,* funded through a variety of programs and aimed at providing a significant research training experience for new doctoral-level scientists and physicians, for those more advanced in their training, for senior-faculty "retraining" sabbaticals, and for promising young MS-dedicated faculty fellows.

In 1992, NMSS allocated $10.6 million to support over 250 separate programs in the United States and abroad. Since NMSS's inception in 1946, over $130 million has been allocated to research and training programs.

MEDICAL PROGRAMS

NMSS is advised by a group of senior medical and scientific volunteers who provide input to staff on a variety of medical-related issues. A Medical Advisory Board of more than 60 active and senior honorary members provides input on a regular or ad hoc basis. Among the Medical Advisory Board's activities are

- *Professional education,* providing staff with assistance in developing written materials and public programs of education concerning MS for physicians, allied health professionals, and the lay public. NMSS sponsors an Issues Forum at the annual meeting of the American Academy of Neurology, works to place MS-relevant keynote speakers at national meetings of other relevant professional associations, and organizes and supports regular international scientific workshops exploring in depth one or more basic or applied research concerns related to the disease.

- *Clinical trials and therapeutic claims,* providing help in evaluating and monitoring studies of safety and efficacy of new therapeutics.

- *Clinic computerization,* providing advice on the standardized collection of MS clinical data in North America on the NMSS/ Canadian MS Society–sponsored MS-COSTAR Computer System.

In addition to these activities, the Medical Advisory Board and its committees provide as-needed assistance with special emergent issues, such as developing guidelines for the use of magnetic resonance imaging in diagnosing MS, development of clinical practice guidelines, and developing core batteries of cognitive function for MS.

SERVICES

Although NMSS does not provide direct financial assistance to people with MS, it does support a variety of service programs to meet the wide-ranging needs of clients with MS and their families.

NMSS's national office houses a substantial Information Resource Center and Library staffed by a team of librarians, social workers, and nurses who respond to more than 3,000 inquiries a month on every conceivable medical and scientific question related to MS. Although not providing medical advice, the center is a needed source of information and referral for clients from around the country who have access to well-advertised toll-free telephone lines.

Most inquirers are served by a staff member who provides immediate information on the phone, and virtually all inquirers receive a packet of information, either general or tailored to a specific request. Each information packet refers the inquirer to his or her local NMSS chapter, where additional information and local services are available.

NMSS chapters are the primary community resource for people with MS. Staffed by fund-raisers, information specialists, and service coordinators and advised by a medical and allied professional advisory committee, chapters regularly survey community needs and resources and aim to fill gaps in service provision at the local level. Among the programs a chapter may provide are support groups, programs for newly diagnosed patients, programs for MS family members and children of MS patients, respite care programs, education symposia for lay and professional audiences, exercise programs (including aquatic therapy), and equipment assistance, as well as individual referral, advocacy, and counseling.

PUBLIC AFFAIRS

To help support its programs of research and services, NMSS conducts a broad range of public awareness programs to familiarize the public with MS; its medical, social, and economic consequences; and the organization's activities. Through a comprehensive outreach, including press conferences, public service announcements in print and broadcast media, and other appropriate activities, the message about MS is carried to virtually every corner of the United States.

Public affairs staff and volunteers also coordinate a significant lobbying effort at the federal and state levels. Working alone or in coalition with related organizations, NMSS works to develop and promote public policy that serves the needs of its membership and to increase funds for research at NIH and related federal agencies involved in health and rehabilitation research. Considerable effort has been expended in recent years to alter Social Security entitlement for disability insurance, to lobby for the 1990 Americans with Disabilities Act, and to formulate a national position on long-term care. Increasingly, state lobbying efforts are becoming important, with local chapters in certain states banding together into a cohesive lobbying force.

PERSPECTIVE ON THE PAST: FUTURE DIRECTIONS

In the United States and many other countries, the needs and concerns of constituents with unique health-related problems have long been served by nonprofit voluntary health agencies and foundations, which can focus on the special needs of a limited population. Such organizations (and in the United States there are almost as many separate organizations as there are diseases) have been instrumental in raising public awareness about special or general health concerns, in shaping public policy, and in providing vital service and research programs that might otherwise go unsupported. The enormous growth of such organizations and their prominence in virtually every sphere of life attests to their need and their success.

In future years, special research and service needs will continue to be served by such specialty organizations, and, as the competition for federal dollars becomes tighter, the role of such health agency programs will become more and more essential.

The future will assuredly bring a need for closer collaboration among health agencies, as key social issues that bridge the interests of separate agencies become more prominent. These issues include major changes in our understanding of the biomedical basis of diseases, which points more and more to the need for collaboration among agencies that deal with similar problems (e.g., immunological disorders). Improvements in medical management that prolong life and contribute to the aging of a disabled population will result in a need for increased collaboration on issues like long-term care, respite services, and needs of caregivers. Finally, current social issues relating to insurance coverage and a spectrum of entitlement programs will become more problematic and will require greater cooperation among agencies to create a louder "voice."

The power of voluntary health agencies to support research and service programs of benefit to their constituents depends, in the long run, on *numbers* of affected people; the challenge for the future will be for agencies to retain individual identity and engage in productive and healthy competition for publicly raised funds, while fostering greater cooperation on those programs and activities of mutual benefit.

For further information on MS and NMSS, consult a local phone directory or call or write to

National Multiple Sclerosis Society
733 Third Avenue
New York, NY 10017-3288
1-800-LEARN MS

Chapter 9

Multiple Sclerosis: A Neurostructural Model of Affective and Cognitive Disorders

Uriel Halbreich, M.D.

The fast-paced and fascinating accumulation of knowledge on multiple sclerosis (MS) illuminates and emphasizes that we are already in the midst of a shift from a descriptive approach to neuropsychiatric disorders to a substantiated understanding of brain pathophysiological processes. For over a century, it has been recognized that affective and cognitive symptoms are quite prevalent in MS. Charcot (1877) described "mental depression similar to classic forms," "foolish laughter without cause," and "stupid indifference" in patients with the disease. Moreover, a temporal association between exacerbations of MS and changes in mood and cognition was noticed by early observers. Even though some symptoms might be reactive to being sick, at present there is no doubt that the main phenomenology is a direct manifestation of the pathophysiological processes of MS. Specific symptoms might be related to specific locations of the pathological defect, even though there are reports that severe affective and cognitive symptoms are more prevalent among patients with widespread nonspecific cerebral involvement as opposed to patients with spinal cord involvement (Rabins et al. 1986; Rao and Leo 1988; Schiffer et al. 1983; Whitlock and Siskind 1980). In such cases it is still unclear whether the symptoms are related to magnitude of spread of lesions and involvement of the central nervous system (CNS) or to impairment in specific locations.

The notion that the symptoms of MS are a consequence of structural change in the CNS, however, is already established. At present, the main questions to be asked are, Where are the abnormal locations? and How and why are these localized lesions formed?

DIAGNOSIS VERSUS DIFFERENTIAL DIAGNOSIS

The emphasize on "where, how, and why" is of generalized importance, because it is quite well accepted (or should be accepted) that cognitive and affective symptoms might be of heterogeneous etiology and constitute the end result of several pathophysiological pathways. Hence, the answer to "What are the symptoms and signs?" does not necessarily provide a definite, clinically relevant answer. Much more is needed for arrival at a diagnosis. The substantial progress in imaging techniques allows for the increasingly refined evaluation of the locations of specific lesions and the association between specific location of pathological process in the brain (which might be one of the symptoms' forming processes) and specific impairment in cognition and emotions. Advances in molecular biology, genetics, immunology, and the biochemical and physiological spheres might provide the answers to "why" and "how." More integrative approaches will answer "why now."

Because MS is usually a disseminated disorder, one might compare location of lesions of patients who have specific symptoms to those who do not present with them. Such an approach can also be applied for evaluation of similarities and differences among a group of disseminated disorders and other neurostructural disorders in which affective symptomatology is prevalent and the specificity of distinct localized lesions as symptoms provoking can be evaluated.

MS and other neurostructural disorders may be used to demonstrate that, as is the general rule in medicine, the description of phenomena (symptoms and signs) is only the first step in the formulation of a differential diagnosis. This process includes information and considerations of the patient's history and the time course of his or her illness, as well as past and present treatment responses. The family history might give some clues to the possibility of genetic susceptibility. The possible temporal association between onset of the disorder or exacerbations of its episodes and distress or traumatic life events might give additional indications for the differential diagnosis. Geographic and environmental contributions might be of significance for some disorders. As is the case with MS, these contributions might not only help in the evaluation of the differential diagnosis, they can also lead to elucidation of the contributing pathological factors.

All these variables are factors in the formulation and evaluation of the differential diagnosis. As discussed in other chapters of this volume, the next step in the evaluation of a patient with suspected MS, or any other neurostructural disorder, is the performance of diagnostic procedures, especially imaging, mostly to assess "where" and "what" is the distribution of lesions. Then laboratory tests should be performed to try to answer "how and why" lesions have developed in the individual being evaluated. The actual diagnosis should be based on etiology and pathophysiology with knowledge of genetics and vulnerability factors. These variables are also the basis for efficacious treatment modalities.

The topics of phenomenology, suggested etiology, and pathophysiology, as well as vulnerability and treatment modalities of MS have been elucidated in previous chapters. In this chapter, I describe examples of other diagnostic entities (or pseudodiagnostic entities) and present the case for generalization.

SYNDROMES VERSUS ETIOLOGICALLY BASED DIAGNOSES

The process of differential diagnosis starts prior to focusing on the possibility of a neurostructural disorder. Same-presenting symptoms or syndromes can be the result of a very wide range of physiological and structural disorders. Some of them are even not initiated in the brain, as can be demonstrated with the evaluation of delirium.

Delirium is a very prevalent condition (Engel 1966; Lipowski 1980) that is currently considered a bona fide DSM-III-R diagnosis (American Psychiatric Association 1987). However, like many other current diagnostic entities, it is actually a phenomenology-based description of a diversified cluster of symptoms and signs that constitute a syndrome or a group of syndromes. These syndromes might be caused by a myriad of pathological processes (Wise 1987), some of them physiological and some of them structural in nature. Therefore, delirium (or "encephalopathy," if a more neurological term is to be used) should be a step in the process of differential diagnosis and not an end point by itself, as might be denoted by defining it as a diagnostic entity. The clustered symptoms of delirium (e.g., reduced level of consciousness, disorientation, impaired perception and cognition, altered psychomotor activity, and disorganized thinking), occurring and fluctuating over a short period of time, raise the possibility of numerous neurophysiological disorders such as alcohol and drug withdrawal, acute metabolic abnormal processes (e.g., hepatic encephalopathy, renal encephalopathy, acidosis, and alkalosis), acute endocrinopathies (e.g., hypo- and hyperglycemia), drug and metal intoxications, infections, postoperative decompensation, and many other pathophysiological processes. It can also be caused by neurostructural localized and (mostly) disseminated pathological processes such as tumors, stroke, abscesses, and hemorrhage.

Indeed, the "real" diagnosis should be the one based on etiology and pathophysiology and not on the phenomenology, per se. Specific treatment is preferably indicated based on the specific etiology. Otherwise intervention is many times merely palliative, adjunct, or supportive.

An important principle that can be demonstrated with the assessment of delirium syndromes is the contribution of premorbid risk factors to the pathophysiology of symptom development. The risk factors include advanced age (but also very young children), cardiotomy, severe burns, drug addiction, and preexisting brain damage (Wise 1987). A conceptual model involving a decrease of threshold for surfacing of symptoms caused by a physical or environmental stressor that affects a vulnerable person has been proposed (Wise 1987).

In summary, the syndromic cluster(s) of delirium might exemplify a final common pathway of myriad of neurostructural and neurophysiological disorders. Different etiological processes might be manifested with the same symptoms. Even when a clear pathophysiological process is demonstrated, predisposing and environmental factors should be taken into account.

RHEUMATIC BRAIN DISEASE

Neurostructural disorders should sometimes be considered etiological factors in the evaluation of many prevalent current nosological entities. The situation is more intriguing not only because that same disseminated neurostructural disorder (DNSD) might be manifested with diversified phenomena, but also because the symptoms might differ according to age at onset or age during a specific episode. The following example demonstrates not only that a specific symptom might be the end result of diversified pathophysiological processes, but also that the same pathophysiological process might be manifested as very diversified symptoms.

In many cases of rheumatic fever, there might be a chronic involvement of the brain. As a consequence, disseminated, unstable, and transient neurological and psychiatric symptoms might appear (Halbreich et al. 1976). Even though rheumatic diseases are disseminated and might affect various organs in the body, the involvement of the CNS is most times ignored. Chorea minor is the only cerebral involvement that is quite frequently diagnosed. The lack of awareness of the possibility of chronic brain involvement in rheumatic cases, and especially in rheumatic fever, is probably the main reason for the infrequency of diagnosis of rheumatic brain disease (RBD) in Western psychiatric literature. In the few early reports on RBD (Bruetsch 1940; Kernohan et al. 1939), rheumatic heart disease was found in 9% of hospitalized patients (diagnosed as having "dementia praecox") and in 5% of autopsies performed on such psychiatric patients. This is in comparison to a prevalence of 1% in the general population of the United States during the same period (Bruetsch 1940; Kernohan et al. 1939).

On the other hand, 3%–12% of patients with a history of rheumatic heart disease had late brain symptoms, usually repeated transient exacerbations of neurological symptoms, with no demonstrated neurological deficit during remissions (Bruetsch 1957; Hutchinson and Stock 1963). At that time, investigators reporting in Russian literature paid more in-depth attention to CNS manifestations of rheumatic processes (Alimov 1973; Chistovich 1963; Fokin 1963; Goldelman 1963; Kushelev 1973; Perervina et al. 1963;

Zimina 1964). Based on that literature, as well as on clinical experience (Halbreich et al. 1976), RBD has been proposed as a distinct entity. The pathophysiology of the disorder stems from disseminated, recurrent rheumatic obliterating arteritis, mainly in small meningeal and cortical vessels. Perivascular and diffuse round cell infiltration has also been described. In some cases (up to 14%) (Halbreich et al. 1976), the CNS symptoms are the result of microinfarcts caused by emboli to small vessels.

The phenomenology of RBD depends on the location(s) of the lesion(s), the patient's age, and the age at onset of the disorder. With this entity, the influence of age on phenomenology of disseminated brain disorders can be well demonstrated. It has been reported (Bruetsch 1940; Kernohan et al. 1939) that when RBD starts at an early age, psychotic symptoms dominate the scene. Acutely there are schizophrenia-like symptoms with acute confusion, hallucinations, and paranoid ideation associated with mild catatonia. Then a personality change of organic type develops with slow evolvement of cognitive impairment, aggression, and impulsive behavior, then followed by a "flat" expression. The need for a differential diagnosis from "idiopathic" schizophrenia is apparent. However, when the same pathophysiological process takes place with a middle-age onset, the main symptoms are "neurosis," anxiety, and depression (Goldelman 1963), with some subtle neurological signs. Later-age onset is manifested mostly with acute psychotic depression, agitation, and rapid dementia, as well as more prominent neurovascular instability and vestibular symptoms (Alimov 1973; Fokin 1963; Halbreich et al. 1976; Perervina et al. 1963). In middle-age and later-age onset, localized neurological, vegetative, and endocrine symptoms are more prevalent than in early-age onset.

INTERACTION BETWEEN LOCALIZED LESIONS, ABNORMAL NEUROCHEMISTRY, AND IMPAIRED CIRCUITRY

Thus far the emphasis in MS research has been on location of plaques and the pathophysiology that might lead to the formation of these localized lesions. However, brain structures are a substruct for biochemical and physiological activities that are dynamically ever-changing. They keep in equilibrium with each other, as well as with other bodily and external processes.

As such, a strict distinction between neurostructural and neurophysiological disorders indeed cannot be made. However, in an attempt to understand and classify such disorders, one can try to differentiate between what is the main effect and what are simply coeffectors, not-so-relevant effects, or even artifacts. In each specific case, the main effect should be at least initially proposed for the purpose of a viable hypothesis or model building. Obviously, sometimes model building is like sailing in the fringes between the realms of fact and wishful thinking. For the sake of a balanced perspective on the current horizons and as an introductory cautionary statement for the following discussion, Gualtieri's note (1991), should be repeated here: "Psychiatry that is based on etiopathogenesis [in contrast to purely phenomenologic descriptive approach] and on brain maps, has rigors. It is either true or untrue. If it is true, like the frontal lobe hypothesis of dopamine agonists . . . it will lead to somewhere. If it is only a small part of the truth, like the Kindling theory of temporal lobe changes, . . . it will be supplanted before long by a more congenial hypothesis" (p. 122).

The understanding of the symptom formation in MS might be enhanced by examples from other relevant disorders. For example, Gualtieri (1991) described an intriguing example of an interface between several processes: a localized lesion that might interfere with circuitry and brain neurochemistry. He noticed that patients who had acquired lesions of the frontal lobes, especially the orbitomedial surface, had a short attention span, locomotor hyperactivity, distractibility, excitability, impulsive behavior, and behavioral disinhibition. He also noticed the similarity between injury-related lesions and the phenomenology of children with attention-deficit hyperactivity disorder (ADHD). Because of the efficacy of stimulants like methylphenidate and dextroamphetamine, as well as the monoamine oxidase inhibitor deprenyl, in treating ADHD, Gualtieri (1991) proposed a hypothesis of impairment of ascending dopaminergic neurons connecting the corpus callosum and the frontal cortex. The same drugs were shown by positron-emission tomography (PET) to improve the hypometabolism in both the frontal lobe and the crpus striatum of patients with ADHD. If these two lines of evidence are true, their convergence is justified. Then we are facing a disorder that can be characterized as being neurostructural *and* neurochemical.

Gualtieri (1991) also claimed that ADHD is an example of localized, specific drug action, but that the dopamine agonists used influence all the dopaminergic pathways in the CNS, including, but not limited to, those that are putatively involved in the disorder described. Therefore they are not specific "frontal lobe medications." Of course, even an attractive hypothesis can not be pushed too far. Nonetheless, the involvement of the dopaminergic system in maintenance of homeostasis has been proposed. In the same way, the role of the frontal lobe as an allassostatic (stabilizing) organ was proposed (Luria 1973, cited by Gualtieri [1991]). Whether the two processes are related to each other or are even key factors in maintenance of homeostasis remains to be proven.

A similar case might be presented for temporal lobe lesions. These lesions are associated with epilepsy but also with psychotic episodes, anxiety states, depression, putatively specific personality patterns, distortion of perception, and exaggerated emotional reactions (Gualtieri 1991). The anticonvulsants and mood stabilizers carbamazepine and valproic acid have been shown to be effective in treating these conditions, as well as bipolar disorders. It has been claimed that these medications might be "temporal lobe drugs." I believe that this is probably not accurate and that their pharmacological action is broader and not location specific. However, the concept of location-oriented medications cannot be dismissed and eventually such medications will probably be materialized.

That lesions in crucial crossroads, points, or end-of-the-road stations of the brain circuitry network might impair the function of that entire particular circuit is very plausible. Along the same line of reasoning, strategically localized lesions might interfere with physiological and/or biochemical connections and information transportation systems in the CNS. Thus the actual distinction between the role of localized structural lesions, impaired circuitry, and physiochemical abnormalities as symptom-forming processes might be blurred.

ARE THERE LOCATION-SPECIFIC SYNDROMES?

Even though current nomenclature defines affective disorders mostly according to their phenomenology and course of illness, it is argued that depressions are a dimension that might be presented across diversified diagnoses. Therefore, depression might be a final result of numerous and diversified pathophysiological processes or a biologically determined abnormality that might be triggered by distinctly different mechanisms. Depressions have been reported to be highly prevalent in patients with various neurostructural disorders. This is probably a manifestation of the abnormality, per se, and not a nonspecific reaction to being sick.

In addition to MS, several other structural disorders have been reported to cause major depressive disorders (e.g., space-occupying lesions, mostly in the frontal lobe; low-pressure hydrocephalus; collagen diseases, such as systemic lupus erythematosus or RBD; Huntington's disease; and stroke in the left hemisphere). Attempts at pinpointing a CNS location or locations associated with depressive mood have not been successful so far. Probably the closest we have come to neuroanatomical localization is in the case of acute stroke. In a 2-year study (Robinson et al. 1985), patients with stroke in the left hemisphere had more prevalent and more severe depressions than those with stroke in the right hemisphere. This finding might be interpreted as suggesting that depression is caused by interference with a circuitry process or neurophysiological process that involves the left hemisphere but not necessarily as pointing to a specific location within this side of the brain.

The perception of depressive mood as a result of multiple and diversified processes inside and outside the brain might exclude a search for a specific location for depression. However, specific symptoms that constitute the phenomenological diversity of affective disorders might be linked to specific brain locations and/ or brain biochemistry. Simultaneously, depression or its severity might be related to the magnitude and spread of generalized structural involvement of the brain (see Chapter 3).

Although depressive mood in general is probably not location specific, other mood and cognitive symptoms are. It has been repeatedly demonstrated that symptom profiles of several neurostructural disorders might be similar to each other. For example, MS, Parkinson's disease, Huntington's disease, and progressive supranuclear palsy (which are sometimes called "subcortical dementias") were shown to present a similar profile of cognitive impairment—mostly in recent memory, conceptual and abstract reasoning, sustained attention, information processing and retrieval, verbal fluency, and visuospatial skills. On the other hand, immediate memory and general intellectual functions are more preserved (Rao 1990, see also Chapter 3). This pattern is different from that of cortical dementias, such as Alzheimer's disease, in which there is mainly an intellectual deficit.

It has been shown that any abnormality of cortical frontal lobe might cause impaired short-term memory storage, concentration, obstruction, problem solving, and judgment, as well as disorientation. Any abnormality of the dominant temporoparietal cortical area might be manifested with impairment of rehearsed consolidated memory; and any impairment of the nondominant temporal cortical area might be manifested by impaired musical memory.

Of intriguing heuristic interest are the suggestions that pathological laughing and weeping in patients with MS might be the result of disconnection of inhibitory circuits involving the brain stem. It has been suggested that a lesion to pathways between diencephalic or brain stem and the right hemisphere frontal lobe might be involved. This might be the ·case with right-handed patients (Sackheim et al. 1982). In patients with stroke, the connections between the pons and the right-middle cerebral hemisphere might be severed (Tatemichi et al. 1987; Yarnell 1987).

The importance of these observations is the possibility of an example of a structural lesion that causes a very specific symptom by interference with brain circuitry. Even though the exact pinpointed location of the lesion might vary somewhat, as long as the lesion is on a specific relevant pathway it might cause the same phenomena.

DIRECTIONS FOR STUDIES OF DNSDs

MS and other DNSDs might be an appropriate model for studies of the association between specific locations of lesions and putative ensuing symptoms. From a methodological view, such studies might be performed in several designs:

1. *Cross-sectional:* Comparison of location and magnitude of lesions in patients who have specific symptoms with those of patients without such symptoms.
2. *Longitudinal:* Comparison of the lesions and symptoms in the same patients during exacerbation, as well as during partial and (if possible) complete remissions. In case of a chronic progressive disorder, both lesions and symptoms can be evaluated at predetermined time intervals. The dependent variables might include a prevalent symptom (e.g., uncontrolled laughing) or a specific prevalent location.
3. *Studies of biological abnormalities with unknown association with the lesions:* In this case, patients with a DNSD, who present with a particular phenomenological syndrome (e.g., major depression), are compared with patients with the same DNSD but without the symptom or syndrome in focus. The biological factors studied are those that are putatively involved in the pathophysiology of the phenomenological syndrome in general. In the case of a syndromic major depression, monoamines' parameters, steroid hormones, peptides, and other factors that were previously studied in patients with major depressive disorder might be studied in DNSD patients with and without depression.

In the above paradigms, phenomenology and biological correlates are better studied across several DNSDs, applying them as a model for involvement of specific processes in the general pathophysiology of the syndrome in focus.

Each and every DNSD differs in the process leading to the formation of the specific localized lesions. The fundamental process might influence brain function and phenomena via biochemical and physiological mechanisms, with no direct location or association to the formation of localized lesions. For instance, in cases of autoimmune disorders or viral diseases, the general "parent" etiological mechanism might start a chain of chemical and endocrine processes that by themselves result in a generalized dysregulation of intraneuronal processes. Similar generalized processes might occur when the original process is vascular or hypertensive. In all these cases, future research is needed to distinguish between phenomena that are location related and those that are process related.

An intriguing phenomenon associated with various neuro-structural disorders is the quite frequent dissociation between a consistent continuous demonstration of lesions by imaging procedures and the fluctuation in clinical status. This phenomenon might add credence to the suggestion that physiological and biochemical processes contribute to symptom formation even in cases of persistent localized lesions. Of special interest are hormonal and stress-environmental influences on the exacerbation of episodes or symptoms. Further elucidation of these variables will hopefully add to our understanding of the intricate relationship between brain structure and function.

As discussed in Chapter 5, treatment-response studies provide fertile ground for the understanding of the pathophysiology of lesion formation. They also provide an opportunity to study the variables influencing symptom formation. The ability to monitor lesions distribution and size over time, in conjunction with follow-up of clinical phenomena and related biological variables, will eventually shed more light not only on the pathophysiology of the specific DNSD in focus, but also on the interaction between structure, physiology, and phenomenology in general.

Indeed the fascinating rapid progress in imaging techniques is continuously opening new opportunities for insight into the brain and its function. The refined ability to study structure *and* function in an increasingly detailed way, as well as the ability to study subtle functional changes over time, will eventually and shortly set the field at a level of applied knowledge unforeseen just a decade ago.

REFERENCES

Alimov KA: Oneiroid syndrome in some acute exogenous organic psychoses. Zh Nevropatol Psikhiatr 73:1208–1213, 1973

American Psychiatric Association: Diagnostic and Statistical Manual of Mental Disorders, 3rd Edition, Revised. Washington, DC, American Psychiatric Association, 1987

Bruetsch WL: Chronic rheumatic brain disease as a possible factor in the causation of some cases of dementia praecox. Am J Psychiatry 97:276–296, 1940

Bruetsch WL: Rheumatic brain disease. Paper presented at the International Congress of Psychiatry, Zurich, Switzerland, 1957

Charcot JM: Lecturers on the diseases of the nervous system delivered at la Salpêtrière. Philadelphia, PA, Henry C Lea, 1877

Chistovich AS: Rheumatic involvement of the brain. Revmatism Revmatoidy 152–165, 1963

Engel GC: Delirium, in Comprehensive Textbook of Psychiatry. Edited by Friedman AM, Kaplan HS. Baltimore, MD, Williams & Wilkins, 1966

Fokin MA: Some features of the vascular tonus in cases of rheumatic lesions of the brain. Vaprosy Revmatisma 3:31–37, 1963

Goldelman MG: Rheumatic affections of the diencephalon. Zh Nevropatol Psikhiatr 63:1445–1448, 1963

Gualtieri CT: The functional neuroanatomy of psychiatric treatments. Psychiatr Clin North Am 14:113–122, 1991

Halbreich U, Assael M, Kawli N, et al: Rheumatic brain disease: a disease in its own right. J Nerv Ment Dis 163:24–28, 1976

Hutchinson EC, Stock JPP: Paroxysmal cerebral ischemia in rheumatic heart disease. Lancet 2:653–656, 1963

Kernohan JW, Woltman HW, Barnes AR: Involvement of the brain associated with endocarditis. Arch Neurol Psychiatry 42:789–809, 1939

Kushelev NP: Pathogenic factors and the anatomical basis of vascular psychoses. Zh Nevropatol Psikhiatr 73:1032–1037, 1973

Lipowski ZG: Delirium: Acute Brain Failure in Man. Springfield, IL, Charles C Thomas, 1980

Luria AR: The frontal lobes and the regulation of behavior, in Psychophysiology of the Frontal Lobes. Edited by Pribram KH, Luria AR. New York, Academic Press, 1973, pp 3–26

Perervina LM, Visgina RI, Shcherback VP, et al: Clinical forms of rheumatic involvement of the nervous system. Aktualnye voprosy Patologii serdechno-sosudistoi sistemy (Kiev) 29–33, 1963

Rabins PV, Brooks BR, O'Donnell P, et al: Structural brain correlates of emotional disorder in multiple sclerosis. Brain 109:585–597, 1986

Rao SM: Multiple sclerosis, in Subcortical Dementia. Edited by Cummings JL. New York, Oxford University Press, New York, 1990, pp 164–180

Rao SM, Leo GJ: Mood disorder in MS. Arch Neurol 45:247–248, 1988

Robinson RG, Starr LB, Lipsey JR, et al: A two-year longitudinal study of poststroke mood disorders: in-hospital prognostic factors associated with six-month outcome. J Nerv Ment Dis 173:221–226, 1985

Sackheim HA, Greenberg MS, Weinman AL, et al: Hemispheric asymmetry in the expression of positive and negative emotions. Arch Neurol 39:210–218, 1982

Schiffer RB, Caine ED, Bamford KA, et al: Depressive episodes in patients with multiple sclerosis. Am J Psychiatry 140:1498–1500, 1983

Tatemichi TK, Nichols FT, Mohr JP: Pathological crying: a pontine pseudobulbar syndrome (abstract). Ann Neurol 22:133, 1987

Whitlock FA, Siskind MM: Depression as a major symptom of multiple sclerosis. J Neurol Neurosurg Psychiatry 43:861–865, 1980

Wise MG: Delirium, in The American Psychiatric Press Textbook of Neuropsychiatry. Edited by Hales RE, Yudofsky SC. Washington, DC, American Psychiatric Press, 1987, pp 89–103

Yarnell PR: Pathological crying localization (abstract). Ann Neurol 22:133, 1987

Zimina ZV: Changes in the CNS in rheumatic carditis. Klin Med (Mosk) 42:60–62, 1964

Index

Page numbers printed in **boldface** *type refer to tables or figures.*